"If there were someone who would try to get a tummy tuck from a skin graft, a rapid weight loss program out of radiation and chemotherapy, liposuction out of a foot reconstruction, and laugh in the face of terminal cancer, it would be Tish Tucker."

—Ike Pauli Jr. M.D.,
Northeast Pediatric Associates,
San Antonio

"*Hear My Cry* will reveal to you how faith and prayer will bring you through the darkest days of your life."

—Elizabeth Travis,
Randy Travis Management,
Santa Fe

"Fascinating yet tempered by humility, honesty, and courage, Tish's intensely personal story is both compelling and intriguing. Diagnosed with an incurable and virile cancer, Tish chose rather to believe in the supernatural healing power of her Lord and Savior, Jesus Christ. Her indomitable spirit is convicting and inspirational."

—Sara S. Abraham,
Executive Director,
Crosses Across America, Inc.,
Vicksburg, Mississippi

"A rare blessing in life is to encounter an individual who inspires you to be better—to yourself, to your family, to friends, and to the community. Tish Tucker comes into one's life as soft as a whisper and shares a heart full of joy, grace, compassion, and courage. She makes the world smile and leaves a little bit of 'forever' in the heart of each person she encounters."

—Annette E. Craven, Ph.D.,
Associate Professor of Management,
University of the Incarnate Word, San Antonio

"Tish's ability to share her personal story reflects her strength and faith in God. Her journey gives resolve, courage, and hope to those whose lives have been touched by cancer."

—Van Mabee,
The Mabee Foundation,
Midland, TX

hear my *Cry*

hear my *Cry*

How grace conquered cancer

Tish Hagee Tucker

TATE PUBLISHING & *Enterprises*

Published by Tate Publishing & Enterprises, LLC
127 E. Trade Center Terrace | Mustang, Oklahoma 73064 USA
1.888.361.9473 | www.tatepublishing.com

Tate Publishing is committed to excellence in the publishing industry. The company reflects the philosophy established by the founders, based on Psalm 68:11,
"The Lord gave the word and great was the company of those who published it."

Book design copyright © 2009 by Tate Publishing, LLC. All rights reserved.
Cover design by Leah LeFlore
Interior design by Nathan Harmony

Published in the United States of America

ISBN: 978-1-60799-070-3
1. Biography & Autobiography: Religious
2. Biography & Autobiography: Medical
09.03.25

Dedication

This book is lovingly dedicated to my husband, Jim, and daughters, Mckenzie and Kassidee, who are my reason for being. To my personal and church families, who offered overwhelming support. And to Rabbi Scheinberg, who prayed for me in stereo. I love you all.

Acknowledgment

I thank God for his mercy and sustaining grace, without which I would not be here today. I am most grateful to the doctors and medical teams at both M.D. Anderson and in San Antonio, who have saved my life and given two girls their mother back, healthy and whole. Words are not enough. Dr. Pauli, we love you so much for allowing us to invade your life and ruin every day off. Thank you for caring for my precious girls! You rock! My love and thanks to my overly-opinionated and outspoken family, who carved out a piece of each day to pray for me and help with my kids. To my Jewish friends across the nation who placed my name before Jehovah God, my deepest thanks. And finally, thanks to Cornerstone Church and the congregations around the world who lifted me up and stood in the gap when I wasn't strong enough to stand by myself. My love and deepest gratitude to you all!

Table of Contents

Foreword

Sooner or later you or someone you dearly love will need a miracle from God to survive. Your urgent need of a miracle may come to you with a phone call from your physician, confirming that your recent medical examination proved conclusively that you have a deadly cancer or life-threatening disease.

Your need of a miracle may come with a knock on the door by a policeman saying one of your children has been involved in a major auto accident and is not expected to live. You walk into the hospital and your beautiful child is a bloody mass of twisted flesh, and you know that without a miracle from God, your child will die.

Your need of a miracle may come when your spouse walks into your bedroom and declares with chilling finality, "I want a divorce!" Fear will seize you by the throat as you feel the dreams of a lifetime slipping through your fingers like fine sand.

Tish Tucker is my daughter! She is married to a wonderful husband with two beautiful daughters, living a wonderful life. Then it happened! A small growth on her right ankle suddenly appeared in a matter of five days, proving to be a leiomyosarcoma—a rare and deadly cancer. When Tish walked through the front door of my home with a medical death sentence over her head, I knew we had to have a major miracle from God.

Tish tells her gripping and life-changing story in her latest book, *Hear My Cry*. It is the story of fears that are faced, realities that are darker than a thousand midnights, and pending tragedy that surrenders to the supernatural triumph we call a miracle.

For you and those you love who are facing the crisis of your life and need a miracle from God, welcome to *Hear My Cry*. Miracles happen! Why shouldn't a miracle happen to you? As you read *Hear My Cry*, begin to expect your miracle. "With men this is impossible; but with God all things are possible" (Matthew 19:26)!

Pastor John C. Hagee
Sr. Pastor Cornerstone Church
San Antonio, Texas

Introduction

In the summer of 2006, I was a thirty-seven-year-old working mother of two beautiful toddler girls when out of the blue, I was diagnosed with a rare and aggressive form of cancer. I was shocked! With no previous health complications, the winds were blown completely out of my sails as I received a terminal cancer diagnosis over the phone while driving down the highway. "You have leiomyosarcoma."

What was I going to do? What was leiomyosarcoma? Where could I turn for help? Was I going to die? I was only thirty-seven! Was my life already over before it really began?

Leiomyosarcoma is a rare sarcoma that affects four out of every one million sarcoma patients. Where could I go to receive world-class medical attention? Would I get it right away, or would I have to wait to be seen? Would the treatment work? Would my insurance cover it?

The questions were numerous, and the facts were few. One fact remained. God was in control. He was not surprised by my circumstances like I was. He knew my end from the very beginning. I prayed that my end would not come soon.

I wanted to be healed, to live a long and prosperous life with my children. I was not going down without a fight.

I gathered my family and friends to surround me with support and prayer regarding every aspect of my life. Extremely independent by nature, I would soon be incapacitated and counting on those around me to perform even the smallest tasks, something I had never before been familiar with ... asking for daily help.

I began to entrench myself in cancer research and literature as well as intense daily Bible studies. I read books that spoke about meditation and finding a "happy place" during treatment. Those books were completed by a family member *after* the author passed away. I did not want someone else to finish my book, so I threw away the ridiculous literature that gave little hope or joy to a weary soul. I concentrated 100 percent on the Word of God, knowing that his promises always ring true.

To say that God was faithful every step of the way is like saying the Pacific Ocean has a few drops of water in it. I was blessed so often and so unexpectedly that I was completely overwhelmed by God's mercy and grace. It was this grace that certainly conquered my cancer.

Every need I had was not only met but exceeded. The love I received from around the world blew me away even more than the cancer diagnosis itself. The miracles that surrounded my healing constantly amazed me, and before long I would hear the words *cancer free*.

If you have ever gone through a life-changing crisis like cancer or stared a daunting enemy in the face, this book is for you. If you know of someone who needs encouragement as they struggle through life's trials, this book is for them. If you have a friend who needs a reminder of how great God is and how precious and fleeting life can be, send this book their way. I pray that God uses this book to transform your life and the lives of your loved ones as you turn the pages. This experience has forever changed me from the inside out, and I wouldn't trade it for the world.

A Deadly Diagnosis

The news was unbelievable. My all-time favorite Pomeranian, Duke, was riddled with cancer at the ripe old age of eight. He had come into my life quite by accident—when the family that owned him couldn't care for his broken leg due to travel obligations. Since that day Duke had been a one-woman dog. He was my child when I didn't have children, and now I was faced with the ultimate dog owner's decision. Specialists were contacted, and there was nothing medical science could do to save his tiny, eight-pound life.

Today was the day I would have to release Duke to where I always hoped he would eventually be waiting for me, Doggy Heaven. It just seemed too soon. There had been no warning signs. One day Duke was sitting on my lap, happy and healthy, wagging his little tail and licking my cheek. The next he was very sick and unable to eat. Dr. Corder, the world's greatest vet, presented me with the daunting news that Duke was not going to recover from this illness.

The sadness surrounding Duke's passing cloaked our house in a way I had not anticipated. His absence penetrated every room. My two girls, Mckenzie (five) and Kassidee (three), were missing him in that innocent way only young children can express. The other two dogs that grew up with Duke moped around the house looking for him and cried when they saw his favorite spots empty. I cried along with them. Yes, we knew he was only a dog, but he had been *our* dog, and he was a very special little guy that had touched each of us in his own special way.

At thirty-seven years old, I was working full-time as a home loan officer, volunteering for multiple non-profit organizations, rescuing animals, and living for the weekends when I could spend quality time with my girls. Crazy was the perfect adjective for our schedules during the week, so every weekend was a golden opportunity to relish the time our children were young enough to think we are brilliant.

My husband, Jim, and I made it our goal to have fun and plan family activities that would interest even the smallest members. This might include mentoring orphans, going to the movies, or helping a local animal shelter, but the girls would always accompany Jim and me so they could understand the importance of family as well as giving back to the community.

On this particular Saturday, the girls and I were looking for something completely frivolous and self-indulgent to lift our spirits. We had just lost our beloved Duke and needed to mourn his passing before returning to work at the shelters. The nail salon was the perfect decadent diversion. While my daughters were enjoying the rhinestone appliqués and bright blue polish, I was enjoying the leg massage and trying not to think about the tiny ball of fluff I would never see again.

This would be my last pedicure for more than a year, as

my world would be violently shaken to the core in just a few short days. The sadness I felt for my dog's passing would be quickly brushed aside in an all-out fight for my own life. One of life's great ironies was about to consume me.

A few days after visiting the nail salon, we attended a baby shower for my sister, Sandy. Family gatherings are always filled with delicious food and familiar faces, like a family reunion but without the crazy relatives you don't like. One face that was unfamiliar to me was David, a lawyer from Washington, D.C.

My dad pastors a church in San Antonio, Texas, with more than twenty thousand members, so it is not uncommon to see new faces at his house, especially during a party. I thought nothing of it as dad introduced me to David. I took sixty seconds to shake David's hand before kissing everyone goodnight and heading home.

I had no idea the enormous and immediate impact David would have on my life, or the role this virtual stranger would play in directing my pre-destined path. I only knew that David was a welcomed guest in our home during an intimate family gathering, so this meant he was an extension of my family.

You know what they say about family…you can pick your friends, but you can't pick your family. All in all, I would say I came out pretty good in the family department. We are a loud group with lots of opinions, but at the end of the day, we are generally supportive of one another, especially during a time of crisis.

And why shouldn't we be? God has blessed us with many things, such as good health, great friends, and happy children. And if God has so graciously bestowed good health on us, we would be remiss to not thank him for it. Health is a gift, something not to be taken for granted, though we are often too stubborn to take the time to attend to our physical needs until they are severe or painful.

Dr. Pauli, our beloved family pediatrician, is the only doctor we see regularly. The adults in my family will call him for advice before waiting in a doctor's office or emergency room. As a general rule, I try to avoid the monotonous waiting that is invariably a part of any doctor's visit. There is no magazine entertaining enough to make me want to sit on a not-so-padded chair for more than fifteen minutes in a waiting room.

However, in April of 2006, my chronically-patient husband had other ideas for me. After a month of severe bronchitis, Jim insisted I go see the doctor. Obviously my coughing was keeping him up at night, so I went to the doctor (under much duress) only to placate my husband. Like every other cough, I knew it would eventually go away if I ignored it long enough.

It had been almost three years since my last checkup, and for my husband to take me to any kind of appointment was an absolute first in eight years of marriage. It's not that I minded my husband going with me, I just assumed he had other things to do. Since my leg wasn't broken, I could very well drive myself. Of course, Jim knew the odds of my not going to the doctor that particular day were great if he did not escort me. So there we were, driving together to the doctor's office with me huffing and puffing all the way.

As we arrived at the doctor's office, the receptionist started laughing as she blew the dust off my file and updated my insurance information. The doctor confirmed the bronchitis, and I was on my way out the door and back to my life when my normally silent husband decided to speak up.

"While we're here, will you check this bump on my wife's right ankle?"

I started rolling my eyes. I wanted to ask him, "Who invited you to this appointment anyway?"

We have several doctors in my family (both certified medical doctors and those who just think they are doctors because they watch late night TV and surf the Internet), and everyone agreed it was probably a ganglion cyst. I glared at my husband, unhappy about having to wait even longer in a doctor's office than was absolutely necessary.

The doctor graciously offered to drain the cyst if I was up for it, so I told him to grab his biggest needle and get on with it. I knew I was stuck in his office until my husband was satisfied, so I decided I might as well make the most of it.

I assumed the time spent on my "cyst" would be minimal, but I was wrong. Doctors can't just start testing; they have to ask you a thousand questions first. I didn't want to answer questions; I just wanted to get back to work. And thus the question and answer session began. How long had the bump been on my ankle? When did I notice it? Was it painful? Had I run into something? Did I fall?

There was no great mystery behind the pea-sized bump on my right ankle next to my ankle bone. The morning after the pedicure with my daughters, this inauspicious bump had appeared out of nowhere. I barely noticed it myself and was shocked to find my husband pointing it out in the doctor's office. First of all, this was a man who rarely spoke in public around strangers unless he was spoken to first. And secondly, he was a red-blooded American male who typically only noticed the radical changes like shaving my head or when his lazy-boy got removed from his favorite spot in the living room to the driveway for the Goodwill truck.

I was both surprised and irritated that he had taken this particular opportunity to notice a tiny bump on my ankle. Of all times, why now? Assuming I had bumped myself on the coffee table or some other piece of furniture, I wasn't really worried about it, as I tend to bruise easily. It wasn't painful, and I really was just waiting for it to dissolve. There was no reason to call Matlock. It was a simple cyst that would fade away in time.

The doctor brought in several different needles and tried to manipulate the cyst and drain it. It wasn't budging. No liquid was draining. We both pushed on the cyst long and hard enough to cause visible bruising when the doctor recommended watching it for a few days to see if it imploded on its own. I was told to call on Monday if the cyst was still intact after the weekend.

Other than the bronchitis, I felt great. No alarm bells were going off in my brain. On Monday I nonchalantly called the doctor back and left a message that the stubborn little cyst was still there and had not dissolved on its own. The recommendation quickly came back for a local podiatrist to observe and possibly remove the cyst. Easy enough. If this would get rid of the bump on my ankle and make my husband happy, then make the appointment and let's move on.

Two days later I was in the podiatrist's office, receiving my second official diagnosis of a ganglion cyst and answering the same set of questions all over again. The podiatrist made another attempt to drain the bruised and slightly swollen knot with several needles, but, just as before, the thick mass was not moving or yielding any liquid.

Unlike the last trip to the doctor's office, my foot was not deadened at all, and I felt like my brain was being pierced with each puncture of the needle stabbing through my foot. At this moment I was not at all happy with my husband and his hot pursuit of the cyst on my ankle. I was daydreaming of poking him with a long needle to see how he liked it. My usually friendly nature was diminishing at a rapid pace.

It was time to move past this constant poking, as the needles weren't yielding any results but tremendous pain. X-rays were taken, and I agreed to get an MRI of the area to verify the cyst theory. I would try just about anything to stop the podiatrist from stabbing me over and over again with various needles and coming up empty. Surely Chinese water torture would render less pain than this relentless plundering of the needle.

The MRI came back showing no ganglion characteristics. The podiatrist insisted it was ganglion, and so did my five hundred friends and relatives whom I'd polled who had absolutely no medical training whatsoever. After three more visits to the podiatrist's office, I decided to have the cyst removed to placate the peanut gallery.

If I really wanted to know what was inside the cyst, then surgery was the only option.

On June 14, my husband drove me to an outpatient clinic in San Antonio. I had never been in the hospital for anything other than the two speedy and flawless births of my girls. No broken bones. No violent allergic reactions. No great emergencies. Nothing exciting to tell on my medical records, which couldn't even fill up a large post-it note.

This surgery was going to be a breeze. It was a non-event, something that needed to be taken care of so I could get back into my favorite strappy heels without an extra bulge on the side of my ankle. I was hoping they wouldn't keep me in recovery too long so I could stop and grab a burger on the way home. I could already smell the jalapeno cheeseburger and fries. As far as I was concerned, I was just doing my husband a favor.

I went in for the nurses to prep me and was handed a generic blue hospital gown as we waited for the doctor to come. These nurses had previously worked with my sister-in-law, Kendal, so they were very kind to me. They treated me like a family member, and I was grateful they made the wait pass quickly, even though much of the time was spent on hospital paperwork and typing my medical history into the hospital's computer system.

By this time I had memorized my rote lines, and I was hoping the nurses would just hand me the computer keyboard so I could type in my own brief medical history and be done with it. That didn't happen, and thus the inquisition began all over again, quickly determining that I was healthy enough for surgery.

After sixty minutes the surgery was complete, and the nurse handed me a Coke to drink while giving me directions on wrapping the wound. Sixty minutes later I was hopping my way through the parking lot, husband in tow. No crutches. No wheelchair. And fortunately, no feeling in my foot for the moment. I was finally on my way to that delicious jalapeno cheeseburger and fries. Yessss!

Over the next few days, my right foot and ankle were swollen, black, blue, numb, and packed with ice. It was painful and began to look like something out of a horror movie as the days passed, but it was a nice break from housework, laundry, running after kids, and life in general. Even though my leg looked like a cross between a decaying mummy and a misshapen purple and green cactus plant, my husband was waiting on me hand and foot, taking the kids back and forth to school, doing the dishes and laundry, and feeding the dogs.

Church members and friends were bringing over food, and my Vicodin refill was full on the nightstand next to me. I had taken two days off work to relax. Life couldn't get much better.

On Saturday, June 17, my very dear friend Sonnette called with the news that her dad had been diagnosed with cancer. My vacation came to a screeching halt. My heart sank. I was devastated for her.

There were no words to tell her how sorry I was, knowing that cancer is synonymous with death. Previously my only experiences with cancer of the non-canine variety were from a safe distance. I had heard many cancer stories over the years, including those of relatives who had fought the disease when I was much younger and not really able to fully appreciate what was going on.

All I could tell Sonnette was, "I will start praying for you and your family immediately." I could not and did not want to imagine being in her shoes. My dad always says, "God is too loving to be unkind and too wise to make a mistake." I had to believe that was true (Isaiah 38:16).

I had to believe that Sonnette's dad was strong enough to pull through, even though he was facing an unforgiving disease. I had thought losing my dog to cancer was horrible, but watching the torture my friend was going through just thinking about her father's immediate future was far worse.

By Monday, June 19, I was on the road again. My husband was chauffeuring me around town in my Suburban, as I was unable to drive so soon after my surgery. My right foot was still swollen, though slightly less horrific. It was still bruised and unable to bend to move the car pedals. So I took advantage of my live-in driver when I needed to get to work, take my kids to day care, or attend appointments.

I had started to like the idea of having a personal driver and felt like a celebrity. "Home, James!" It was great. I could accomplish so much while I was sitting on the highway when I didn't have to worry about driving.

Just as I was patting myself on the back for my multitasking skills on the drive to pick up my kids, my cell phone rang. The podiatrist was on the other end, and he very quickly said, "I know you are coming in for a checkup tomorrow, but I wanted to tell you that the tests results came back from pathology, and you have leiomyosarcoma."

That was the last thing I heard. My lips kept moving, and words were coming out of my mouth as I continued asking questions, but my brain was somewhere else entirely, frozen in time. My head was swimming in a dense fog of unanswered questions and horror. In one single breath, I had been handed a death sentence.

Shock and disbelief permeated my very being. I was in my own episode of *The Twilight Zone*. It was a total out of body experience where I was having a conversation with myself that made absolutely no sense while everything else in my universe ceased to exist. Everything around me went completely black, though I did not lose consciousness. All time and space were instantly suspended as this unexpected diagnosis hit me full force.

Did he just say I have a sarcoma? Sarcoma is cancer. And what was the first part he said? What kind of sarcoma? Did they mix up the test results? Surely this can't be right. I better write it down. Maybe the pathologist got it wrong. People who get cancer die*! My dog just died of cancer. Was he really talking to* me*? Did he read the wrong chart? Did he dial the wrong number? He's not an oncologist. I'm not a smoker. How could I have cancer? I might eat too many candy bars, but that wouldn't give me cancer. Would it? Maybe I should start jogging. Did he just tell* me, *I have cancer? There is no way I could have cancer. A month ago this bump wasn't even on my leg, and I'm not in any pain. Everyone said it was a ganglion cyst. It can't be cancer! He can't be talking about me. I'm only thirty-seven! Maybe he missed that day in cancer school. I'm healthy. I look great. I feel great. I'm really young and very active. I don't have time for this. I have a ganglion cyst. They are looking at the wrong medical chart. I can't possibly have cancer. I don't feel sick. I'm just too young to have cancer. This can't be happening to* me*!*

The disjointed conversation inside my head was endless and chaotic. There was no point where it became logical or where any questions were answered. It was all very surreal as I tried to wrap my mind around the fact that I had just been diagnosed with cancer. I, Tish Hagee-Tucker, a thirty-seven-year-old woman with an unscathed health record and two young girls, had just been diagnosed with cancer, a terminal disease, over the phone. Thank God I wasn't driving!

Startling reality was stabbing me repeatedly like a cold knife in my chest. There was no escaping the unexpected, seemingly fatal turn my life had taken with just one phone call. At that moment I had no idea how long or short my life would be. Was I still going to be around when my daughter started kindergarten next year? I was frozen in complete shock, hanging in this alternate universe, having a conversation with myself where words like death, cancer, sarcoma, and no survivors began to cocoon themselves around me.

I suddenly heard a soft but deep voice in the distance. It took me several moments to realize that my conversation with the doctor had ended and my husband was talking to me. "What did the doctor say?" The answer stuck to my tongue like glue as I stumbled through my own disjointed thoughts, trying to choose the right words. Two years before my own diagnosis, Jim's mother died after her own battle with cancer, so I knew this would be especially difficult for him.

There was no way to soften the blow or sugarcoat the news. My brain could not come up with an easy way to relay the fact that I could be dying. All I could do was stare directly down at the legal pad on my lap and read the notes I had jotted sometime during my conversation with the podiatrist. They were random words written in nonsensical circles.

I whispered in an almost inaudible tone, "He said I have leiomyosarcoma."

Jim's voice went deadly still as he softly asked, "Is that a type of cancer?"

I could hear the pain in his voice and wanted to ease his

concern, yet I could not face the reality myself. All I could do was nod as the blood drained from his tanned face. A thick silence punctuated by the unknown consumed us.

Though I had wondered if the doctor had made a mistake, I knew in my heart that the words rang true. I had cancer. The pathologist that confirmed the diagnosis was trained at M.D. Anderson in Houston, Texas, a hospital that is world renowned for its research and treatments of all types of cancer.

They were reading the right chart. No matter how many times I told myself this bit of news, the daunting reality of the situation would not set in. I knew what the doctors were telling me was true, yet it was incredibly hard to accept. It was like having a miscarriage. You know that you are no longer going to have the baby, but you just don't want to believe the facts because they are too painful. Yet the fact remained.

My husband and I were both still in the car, now driving aimlessly down the highway, as the news was too much to discuss in that moment of sensory overload. We both knew that we would sit down and talk about it eventually, but we had to deal with our own emotions first and try to dredge up some semblance of reason from this madness that had so completely captured our attention.

My heart began to ache as I could palpably feel my husband's pain and concern. How many people would cancer cost him? The intense rush of sadness had to be swept away quickly, as I knew I would never be able to pick up my kids without breaking down in front of them. A complete meltdown was not an option, so I began to focus on contacting my immediate family members, so that they could hear this disturbing news straight from the horse's mouth.

The worst part about bad news is sharing it with the ones whom love you the most. My dad says that parents are only as happy as their saddest child. I was definitely going to be the rain cloud on top of our family's picnic. Scratch that, more like Tropical Storm Tish.

There was no way around it. I had to tell my family, because cancer was a demon too large to tackle on my own. I hated telling myself the news. How was I going to tell *them*?

Nothing made sense. I had no idea what to do or even where to begin, so I just sat there, staring blankly at the pad of paper lying in my lap, wondering who I would have to break the news to first.

I felt like the guy in the black car who delivers the news to military wives that their loved one is not returning. I was the driver in the black car in this scenario, but instead of delivering news about someone else, I was forced to deliver this unexpected information about myself. How do you tell a parent that you might be dying? As I began to think of how to word my conversations, random thoughts flooded my senses.

I could hear the words *terminal disease* repeating themselves over and over again in my head, the news reverberating inside and bouncing from one part of my brain to the next like a tiny ping pong ball in a sudden death match. My sense of logic and emotion began to war inside of me in search of the truth. I wanted to call the doctor back and remind him that I was only supposed to be there for my bronchitis.

I did not want anyone to check the ominous box on my chart that said "Cancer." How could I keep up with my two little girls if I had a terminal disease? Who would keep them if I died? How would their lives change? Would they still be able to go to college?

I was not thinking of the numbers of survivors but of those who had lost the battle and the overwhelming number of statistics. I was wondering if my life would be truncated as if it were of no value and wondering why I hadn't done more with the time I had already been given. I was on a roller coaster ride that heightened every emotion in my body and dulled anything remotely related to rational thinking. But, like tiny flurries of snow, as one thought melted away, another one took its place.

I didn't want to hear my days could be numbered and my girls could grow up without a mother. I wanted to celebrate turning forty with my family and friends and continue dying my gray hair every color of the rainbow. I wanted to be old enough to watch my hair fall out for reasons other than chemotherapy. I felt the same as I had the day before, yet everything was completely different.

Random and ridiculous thoughts continued racing through my brain at warp speed as my husband continued to silently creep down the highway. I finally worked up the nerve to call my mom. I thought I would start with, "I'm going to be a little late picking up the kids," and work my way up to, "And by the way I have cancer." But no one answered the phone.

Letting out an exhausted breath, I dialed my dad's number and was oddly relieved when Diana answered the phone. I didn't know if it would make me feel better or worse to share the news with my family, but I knew that this was something they needed to know. After Diana said hello, I quickly began rambling something from the vague notes that were outlined on my pad, and she asked me to come over right away.

While driving to dad's house, I tried calling other family members to give them the news firsthand but was met by several answering machines. I couldn't very well leave a message saying, "Just wanted to let you know I have cancer. Call me later when you have time and we'll do dinner to discuss. Ciao."

I hung up and decided that Diana could make the calls for me. She called my brother, Chris, and he called the next person and so on. We were keeping the news limited to family and very close friends, as we really didn't know the severity or scope of what we were dealing with. And I needed to get a grip on the sudden nose dive my life had taken.

As hard as I tried to put a halt to the non-stop questions that infiltrated my every thought, I knew that the current light at the end of my tunnel was a fast-moving train, and I was stuck on the tracks. My mind continued to drift in every possible direction.

Was the cancer widespread? Would treatment help me? Where could I go for treatment? What if no treatment was available to me and we found it too late? How could I feel so good and have a terminal disease? Was this a kind of cancer I could live with for years? Was I going to die soon?

When I arrived at my dad's house, he was standing on the front steps in his house shoes, sporting an expression I was unfamiliar with. My dad is the kind of person you can hand a million dollar problem to, and he can resolve it in less than five seconds on a slow day. He will say something like, "The federal deficit is a problem. The war in Israel is a problem. What you have is not a problem. All you need to do is …"

Dad preaches a sermon series entitled, "Promise, Problem, Provision." The premise is that God gives you promises in the Bible for every problem you will face in life. For every million dollar problem, there will be a million dollar provision, but you have to seek God's will and stand on his promises to carry you through the problem. Your attitude in the problem will determine how long you stay in the problem.

I certainly had a ten million dollar problem staring me in the face. I was waiting for my dad to hand me the five-second remedy, to tell me he had a ready-made answer for this death sentence that I had just been handed over the phone. His grim face showcased a level of deep concern. One quick look at the stern lines etched around his clenched jaw told me that a five-second answer would not be the case today. There was no soft smile or joke to wash away the problem.

I didn't think it was possible, but my heart sank even deeper. I knew if my dad was concerned, then I was facing a legitimate problem, a viable opponent that would not easily be defeated. Gripping reality began to soak through every pore. Dad was just as shocked as I was. This was certainly uncharted territory for all of us, and a cold numbness began to spiral through my body as I slowly ascended the staircase to his front door.

Dad wrapped his arms around me and said, "Come inside."

My dad is all about getting to the source of the problem, and this would be no exception. Since I had no recollection of my phone conversation from the car other than hearing the word "leiomyosarcoma," he and Diana called the podiatrist right away so they could hear the news firsthand and ask questions.

Dad began filling in the blanks and asking the series of

questions I might have asked if I had been even remotely lucid. He received the same answer to every question. "She needs to see an oncologist, and the sooner the better. I don't have any more details to give you." Having only seen cancer a few times in his career, the podiatrist encouraged us to seek further information from a trained sarcoma specialist.

In retrospect, this was the best advice he could have given, as sarcoma is an animal all its own. Oncologists with special-ized training in sarcomas are the only doctors that should treat sarcoma patients, as sarcomas react differently than other vari-eties of cancer. If a doctor does not see several sarcoma patients each month, he or she is not considered a specialist.

While the podiatrist was talking to my parents, I felt like they were having a conversation about a church member or someone else's mother, daughter, wife, or co-worker, anybody else but me. My father pastors a large church, and the reality is that someone is always sick or dying. But no matter who it is, you never get used to the word cancer. You never want to hear *that* word attached to the name of someone you know or love.

Similarly, you never want to hear that someone's child is dying. Now I was that child. I was the one with the terminal disease. I was the one they were describing as the girl with cancer. The news was very raw and difficult to digest.

Before I left my dad's house that night, he announced in his normal tone of absolute confidence, "We have to turn to the Bible. It has been a good book for us, and God will not fail us now."

And that was it. It was like a switch had turned on inside of me and my boxing gloves were on. I was down but not out

(Psalm 37:23–24). It was time to shake the dust off my shoes and put the smile back on my face.

I could no longer think of my two beautiful, blonde-haired, blue-eyed daughters wearing black dresses and waving goodbye as my coffin was lowered into the ground. I could no longer think of how my husband would be affected by losing another family member to cancer in such a short period of time. I couldn't lament the things I hadn't done or places I hadn't visited. I had to focus 100 percent of my energy on God's Word and how much had been planted in my soul over the past thirty-seven years (Isaiah 40:8). I needed to personify the attitude of gratitude, for I had truly been given far more than I ever deserved.

I was about to watch the seeds that had been planted over almost four decades come into full bloom overnight. We had all been knocked down by the news, but staying down was not an option (Joshua 23:10). As the old saying goes, "quitters never win, and winners never quit."

On my way out the door, Diana warned me to stay away from the Internet, as most of the information available described a slow, painful death with very little hope and a maximum life span of five years after diagnosis. Of course, I needed to know what leiomyosarcoma really was, so I looked up various cancer foundations and found out that leiomyosarcoma is a rare form of cancer that affects four in every one million sarcoma patients.

It spreads through the blood stream and can affect any soft tissue in the body, lungs, liver, or blood vessels. There is no cure, and it can recur anywhere at any time. It can be dormant for more than a decade and come back with a vengeance. Even if treated, leiomyosarcoma can be a silent killer. It is usually undetected until the major organ it has destroyed stops functioning.

I was on a mission to find the truth about what my condition truly was. What was leiomyosarcoma, and how was it going to affect me personally? I needed some answers before my family relayed the news to others. I needed to grasp what was happening to my body before I could deflect anyone else's questions. I needed some kind of direction, a more definitive idea of what was happening to me. It was an enormous pill to swallow that was encapsulated in a thick layer of unknown variables.

On the drive home, I started thinking about how I was going to beat this dreaded cancer that I had just been told about. I was trying to carve a hole out of the thick fog that had infiltrated my brain, freezing all formidable thought processes. I started thanking God for the many blessings in my life, including the amazing support team that I had living in the very same city with me.

In my family, when someone has a problem, we "circle the wagons." This means we circle that person in our prayers and offer every means of physical support until the problem is resolved. One brother or sister calls the next, and we get the message out very quickly. Physical arrangements are made until every need is met.

I have two brothers and two sisters, all of whom are married to great people, all of whom I was relying on to lift me up in prayer. I was in a fight for my life, and I needed all the help I could get.

By the time I arrived at my house, exhaustion had taken

its toll. I said a very quick and simple prayer before going to bed. When I talk to God, I keep it simple and I keep it real. I don't try to pretend like I'm Shakespeare or that God doesn't already know my circumstances. God knows that I am educated, and I don't have to speak in Elizabethan English to prove it (Matthew 14:12–14). As Matthew 7:7–8 says:

> Ask, and it will be given to you; seek, and you will find; knock, and it will be opened to you. For everyone who asks receives, and he who seeks finds, and to him who knocks it will be opened.

I wanted to knock very, very loudly that night so God would know he had my full attention. I wanted him to know I was not like Moses; I wanted to learn whatever he was trying to tell me the very first time. I did not want to be wandering in this cancer wilderness for forty years. I did not even want to be Samuel, who had to be called by God three times before he realized who was talking. *I got it!* I was ready. I wanted to be "all ears" like H. Ross Perot. Whatever God was telling me, I wanted to catch the full meaning on the first lap around the mountain. I did not want to die searching for the Promised Land.

I got down on my knees with my head and ankle throbbing and said, *"God, thank you for this opportunity. I don't know what you want me to do right now or how this will turn out, but I know that you knew the answer before I knew there was a problem. Thank you for trusting me with this cancer. Thank you for allowing me to grow in you. I know you must trust me a lot to give me such a great assignment, so I want you to know that I am listening. I want to hear you the very first time. I don't know how long or difficult this road will be, but I ask that you give me strength for the journey. I'm not asking you to make my journey easier or the road shorter; I'm just asking for you to be with me, to guide me, and to give me your strength, because I simply cannot do this on my own. And I am begging you to please let me live, if this be your will, because I would love to be able to spend the rest of my long life with my two precious little girls whom you gave me. Please don't let them watch their mommy die. In Jesus' name, amen."*

The presence of God in my room after that prayer was so thick and delicious that I could have served it in ice cream bowls with hot fudge on top. God's message was coming in loud and clear. *Do not fear. I am in control. Put your trust in me (Proverbs 3:5). Your healing is only a matter of time. Look to me, the Author and Finisher of your faith (Hebrews 12:2). I am the Alpha and the Omega (Revelation 1:8). Do not look at the circumstances surrounding you, but keep your focus on me. I will carry you through this storm (Matthew 6:33–34).*

This was the message that would be relayed to me time and time again by people from all walks of life in various ways. I knew without a doubt that if I stayed focused on the face of God, I would survive this thunderstorm. I also knew that if I looked around I would surely drown in a sea of fear and doubt.

I was not afraid of dying (Matthew 14:1–3). If I died tomorrow, then I would be going to a place where I could sleep in every day and never pay another bill (John 14:2). No more work, no more laundry, no more dishes, no more chores, no more alarm clocks.

But what about my children? The concern that weighed most heavily on my mind immediately after my diagnosis was, what would happen to my children if I died? Would they eventually blame God for taking me while they were so young? Would they be able to fulfill their own spiritual destinies if I wasn't there to guide them? Would they shun a life of ministry because of my death? Would they reach their full potential, or would they become bitter and full of unforgiveness?

It was an overwhelming day that had sucked the last bit of energy from my mind, body, and soul, so I began to read the Bible and thank God for his answer, which I knew was on the way. The great thing about hitting rock bottom is that you can only go up. In this case, I was looking up for the answer.

God knew how my problem would turn out before I even knew a problem existed. He knew exactly how many days I had left. And if his eye is on the sparrow, I knew he was watching me (Matthew 6:25–34).

Psalm 147:4 says: "He counts the number of the stars; he calls them all by name." If he calls the numerous stars by their individual names, he certainly was aware of my recent circumstances. It was time for my little star to shine and give God the glory for the great things he was about to do in my life.

I immediately fell into a deep sleep and began to dream. I am not Martin Luther King or Joseph, so I do not dream in Technicolor on a regular basis or parade around in a colorful robe. In fact, I am usually asleep before my head hits the pillow because I'm so exhausted after working all day, doing volunteer activities, cleaning up after my pets, and running after two small girls. I merely look at my pillow and start snoring.

For me to dream is unusual. To remember the dream is unheard of. God does not come into my bedroom and write long scrolls on the walls, and I am not a religious fanatic with a secret decoder ring.

My dream began with me driving alone in my Suburban. (At the time I couldn't drive myself because my foot had not yet healed from the surgery, and as a mother I am never alone in the car.) I was driving alone, and my Suburban was totally silent. No TV. No radio. No children. I was driving on a cloverleaf that was dangerously high above the highway, much higher than a normal exit ramp. It was so far above the highway that it seemed I could touch the clouds if I rolled down my car window.

I clearly heard someone telling me to put on my seatbelt. At that very moment, I saw a huge pile of debris in the center of the road. I swerved to miss the debris, and my Suburban flew off the cloverleaf. I was floating in mid air. As I was free falling through the air, waiting to crash, angels came on every side of my Suburban and carried me on their wings until I was safely placed on the highway below. I was perfectly safe, and my car didn't have a scratch.

When I woke up I realized that God's Word would be my seatbelt for the rough road that was surely ahead. He would cover me with his wings and no harm would come to me as long as I looked to him for the answer. This was my golden opportunity to reach out to others who were going through a similar battle, because I knew my healing was just a matter of time.

I had asked for healing. Now it was time to thank him for that healing. I didn't know how, and I didn't know when, but I knew beyond a shadow of a doubt that God had clearly told me I would be healed.

For the next several days I tried to relay my current circumstances to my brain. At one moment I would understand the concept that I had just been diagnosed with cancer, and the next I had to pinch myself to come back and focus on the task at hand. I was constantly floundering between my previous "non-cancerous" universe and this new place I was living: Cancer Land. I did not want to be a citizen there. People would look at me with undisguised sorrow in their eyes as they asked how I was doing. I would smile and give my usual, chipper, "Fine, thanks for asking."

It's like when you first find out you are pregnant. You are really excited, but it just doesn't seem real. Once you hear the heartbeat of the baby growing inside you, it becomes very real. You suddenly understand that you are really going to become an actual non-sleeping, tax-paying parent.

When you are first diagnosed with cancer, it doesn't seem real. There are often no outward signs of cancer, and you don't feel any differently that you did the day before. Until you hear a doctor tell you, then show you actual test results, you can't really grasp the fact that you are harboring a disease that has no cure to date.

At that moment, it would probably have been easier to hear that I had been impregnated with twenty kids after having my tubes tied. The news was just that difficult to understand. And every time I opened my eyes, there it was, staring me in the face.

I had to constantly remind myself that I was the one who had cancer this time. It wasn't a church member or friend, it was *me*. As people would walk by, they would morbidly stare at me like I had grown a third head or was coated in yellow caution tape. They didn't know what to say or how to act.

It was very hard to believe that grown men and women

did not know what to say as I passed by them in the hallway. When I looked in the mirror, I saw the same rosy-cheeked reflection of the same woman who had been there the day before. Yesterday my biggest concern was getting the bills paid on time and feeding the kids something besides Snickers for dinner. Today I was praying that God would allow me to live through several more dinners with my kids.

It was an immediate re-aligning of my priorities. Since my pants covered the surgical casings on my leg, I could not understand the deep sympathy emanating from the eyes of every passerby. I wanted to scream, "I am going to live! No matter what I have to do, or how long it takes, I am going to live!" (Psalm 118:17–18).

The Cross at
My Crossroad

I continued living my life just as I had before, only with a higher intensity of appreciation for even the smallest things. I enjoyed every second I had with my family, every meal we shared together. I wanted to make the most of whatever time I had left. I could not wait to get to church to thank God for revealing the unknown (Daniel 2:22).

That Sunday morning dad gathered the elders of our church in his office, and each of them laid hands on me as they began to collectively pray over me (1 Timothy 4:14–15). These were people I had known most of my life. As a family we had prayed when their kids were sick and dying or when they had been to the hospital, but I never expected to be the one whom everyone was laying hands on because of a terminal disease.

It is easy to ask someone to pray about your job promotion or your finances, your kids at school or finding God's will in your life. It is another thing all together to ask someone to pray that you will be healed so that you can avoid death. The stakes are very high. Unlike not getting the promotion, not being healed has much greater consequences.

So there I was, in the center of a gathering of elders, lifelong friends whom I have known since I actually wore my natural hair color and braces, and I was asking them to pray that my life would somehow be miraculously extended. Having just had a few short days to personally absorb my diagnosis, it was still very surreal for me to grasp the concept that I had just had a cancerous tumor (not a cyst) removed from my body. Even in this intimate setting of family and friends, after several days of absorbing the shock, the questions persisted.

Was there more that the doctors didn't find? Would the cancer spread too far before I found a good sarcoma specialist?

I realized that only God knew the answer to these questions. At that moment the impervious smoke that had engulfed me for days began to dissipate as the realization hit me that I was truly not alone in this fight.

Some of the people laying hands on me were cancer survivors themselves, and that gave me much hope. I was looking around at a circle of winners, a circle of real believers in the unrelenting and miraculous healing power of God! I was surrounded by people who had walked a mile in my shoes and lived to tell about it.

Still, my cancer was very rare, and I had a good idea that things would get much worse for me before they got better. The insatiable uncertainty of what I was dealing with seemed to be growing, but I refused to allow fear to overcome me. I knew that fear and doubt would surely kill me faster than any cancer (2 Timothy 1:7).

After this corporate prayer, Dad preached a sermon he

wrote about healing after learning of my diagnosis. I have heard hundreds of sermons in my life, but that will always be my favorite. It was my sermon.

When we think of God healing us, we think of our physical bodies. But God can heal anything, and he usually works from the inside out. He can heal hearts, homes, marriages, relationships, and he can certainly heal cancer. He is the master of the impossible. He is at his best when we are at our worst. He was not surprised by my cancer like I was. He was not reeling from the reality. He was large and in charge. It was time for me to get a grip.

I quickly came to despise the term cancer victim. I didn't feel like a victim at all. I was not choosing to be a victim. Victims are people who thrive off everyone else's pity. I wanted to be a survivor. I wanted to be a thriver. No matter what happened to my body, mentally I was preparing myself to be victorious. This was a game where the winner takes all, and I couldn't afford to lose.

I had no idea God would use this cancer diagnosis to show me how very special I was to him. I began to drown in God's love in a way that was all-consuming and overwhelming. I had no idea how much I meant to God, and it took cancer to show me (Romans 8:37–39). After all, I was only one person. How much can one person really mean?

My expectations regarding my health were very realistic, even though I was uncertain of what my immediate future would hold. I was absolutely convinced I would need an unprecedented amount of spiritual and emotional strength. I was not trying to kid myself that the road would be easy, because what little I knew of cancer was very ugly indeed.

Cancer is not a respecter of persons. Cancer doesn't care how rich or poor you are, how beautiful or ugly, what a great job you have, or if you are in the middle of a huge project at home. It can lay claim to anyone, anywhere, at any time without rhyme or reason. I have yet to hear of anyone who was expecting to get cancer.

It strikes without warning, wounding with poisonous venom that can saturate your entire being as it destroys your body, heart, and soul. It can tap into the innermost recesses of your mind and take complete control of your emotions. Cancer is an unforgiving demon that can take over your entire life if you allow it just the smallest entrance.

My thought was, *If I do not allow strangers into my home in order to prevent robbery of my physical possessions, why would I allow Satan to use cancer to steal my peace and my joy?* Cancer is a tough tutor that wastes no time. Once you've been diagnosed, you quickly learn what is truly important.

For example, tangible items are not important, but you cannot live a truly successful life without peace and joy. You cannot walk through a storm alone and hope to jumpstart your life in a healthier direction once the thunder and lightning have passed (John 14:27). You need to know that God is on your side, helping you in the middle of the storm, and not just waiting for you safely on the other side. He is there to hand you the life jacket when the seas are tossing you about. Romans 5:1–5 says:

> Therefore, having been justified by faith, we have peace with God through our Lord Jesus Christ, through whom also we have access by faith into this grace in

> which we stand, and rejoice in hope of the glory of God. And not only that, but we also glory in tribulations, knowing that tribulation produces perseverance; and perseverance, character; and character, hope.

I was full of hope and determined to fight every day for the rest of my life if necessary. I was completely exhausted on every physical level. Parts of my leg that I never even knew existed began to hurt. But mentally and spiritually I was stronger than ever. It had been just a few days since my diagnosis, yet it felt like I had aged years.

Where should I go? Whom should I call? Where is the best sarcoma specialist located? How long will it take for someone to see me? Will I have to leave the state or the country for treatment? Will I have to be gone long?

The questions just kept coming, and I really didn't know when they would be answered. My dad decided it was time to take action. He made a call to David in Washington, D.C. Remember the David I met at my sister Sandy's baby shower; the man I shook hands with for five seconds before heading home?

David was about to become my knight in shining armor. Previously he had worked for Senator Arlen Spector, who had appropriated millions of dollars to cancer research, so David graciously volunteered to go to Capitol Hill on my behalf and request information on the very best sarcoma oncologist in the world. He quickly called back and directed us to Dr. Benjamin, who is in charge of the sarcoma department at M.D. Anderson, right down the road from us in Houston. It was indeed a small world after all!

As news of my illness began to slowly penetrate circles outside of my immediate family, people began asking an ungodly amount of questions. For example, why seek the help of medical professionals if I believed in God? I believe God gave us medicine and some of the most gifted doctors on the planet. Why would I waste this most valuable commodity? I was counting on God to put together a medical team of the best physicians for my particular illness, hopefully at M.D. Anderson. This group would be hand-selected by the Great Physician himself for my ultimate healing.

God would receive all the glory, but I was not about to become an ostrich and stick my head in the sand. When you go to war, you load up on weapons. You don't leave the bullets behind.

Denial is not a way to defeat cancer. I wanted to acknowledge the problem and then give it to God, who would in turn assign angels to protect me (Psalm 91:11). Cancer was a burden far too heavy for me to carry alone, so I laid it at the altar and told Jesus that I would need to be carried for a while, because my body and mind were battered and bruised, and I knew that the fight had only just begun (Matthew 11:28–30).

It was time for my life to truly become meaningful. I'm not talking about the philosophical questions that you hear in school like, "Is the chair really there?" I mean the true meaning of life, granted by the Giver of Life. If I was the only one on earth, Jesus would have died just for me. What had I done to be granted a second chance at life? There was no quid pro quo, no reciprocity for the things God had already done in my life. It made me feel so unworthy to think about the enormity of his sacrifice for me.

When I started to think about Jesus carrying me throughout this time of illness, I started to think about the cross and what an astronomical burden that must have been. Yet there was no one else who could have shared in that event without altering the universe as we know it. What did the cross really mean to me at this particular crossroad in my life? I had heard the story thousands of times and could easily recite it in my sleep.

The story of the cross was suddenly very vivid and meaningful to me as I began to think about what heaven might really be like. What would the next life entail (John 14:1–3)? I felt like I could almost touch it at this point, like my San Antonio residency voting card might be expiring in the very near future. No one really knew exactly what turns my disease would take.

The one thing I was certain of: my gratitude for the cross. Without the cross I would have no hope of a future walking on streets of pure gold and opening gates made of pearl on the way to my very own mansion (Revelation 21:21). This would certainly be an upgrade from my current living conditions. If there were no Calvary, then my last breath here on earth would be the end of my story; it would all be over. There would be much to cry about if that were the case.

But Calvary did happen; it was a very tangible story of selfless love that was being played out before my very eyes. Jesus could have said one word, and the cross would have never happened. One word and I would have no hope of surviving cancer. One word and, if the cancer killed me, I would be all dressed up and have nowhere to go.

Honestly, if I had been hanging on the cross for a crime I didn't commit (cancer) and my father told me I was taking on the punishments of everyone around me and that I would ultimately die for something I did not do...I have to say that I would tell him to just forget about it. Let their punishment fit their own crime. Why should I be the one to pay for everyone?

Fortunately for mankind, the Son of God has much more compassion. Jesus, the giver of all good and perfect things, took my sins and my disease on his back (James 1:17). He died a slow and painful death so that I (who have never been anywhere close to perfect) wouldn't have to. Jesus withstood total public humiliation, took my cancer to the cross and died in my place (Hebrews 12:2).

I have been to Israel and walked the narrow cobblestone streets of the Via Dolorosa as they wind their way to the sight of Christ's ultimate sacrifice. I have stood on Golgotha, a relatively small hill when you live close to the Texas hill country. This seemingly inconsequential pile of rock and dirt changed the course of history.

I began to daydream and take myself back to that small Israeli hill that I had visited so many years ago. In my mind's eye I was a spectator on the day that Jesus was crucified. I was a small person on the periphery absorbing the seemingly catastrophic events of the day, suffocating in the emotions that were being played out by various participants. This day of all days seemed to be the worst in human history but ultimately ended up changing the world forever for the better.

Of course, as a spectator I did not know what would happen after the cross. I had no anticipation of Christ's resurrection. I watched in utter disbelief and sadness as I watched the King of Glory get spit upon for crimes he did not commit.

I heard the mocking and bitter curse words of the soldiers

dragging him down the narrow cobblestone streets, where he stumbled many times on the broken rocks used as a rudimentary pavement. I heard the whip cutting through the air and ripping his flesh time and time again as the tiny shards of metal pierced his back. I saw blood dripping down his face from the crown of thorns as he was surrounded by soldiers who offered up resounding laughter at the King of the Jews.

I heard the clang, clang, clang of the hammer as it ripped through bones and flesh, nailing Christ to the Cross between two thieves. I felt a wave of unbearable sadness as the physical pain began to tear away any signs of life from his body. I saw the anticipation in his eyes as the soldier picked up the final spear and rammed it into his side, his body slumping on the cross.

And I felt his mother's salty tears as they stained her face, her heart slamming into her rib cage and shattering into a million pieces at the sight of her child suffering in such an inhumane manner. I understood her sense of total loss and anguish, her feeling of total desperation at not being able to help her only child. And all of this so that the only perfect person who ever walked the earth could save me from my sins and give me an eternal home. He died for *me*. And he died for *you*. Isaiah 53:5 says:

> But He was wounded for our transgressions, He was bruised for our iniquities; The chastisement for our peace was upon Him, and by His stripes we are healed.

What had I done with my life to deserve that kind of selfless love? What had I done to deserve that kind of unequivocal mercy? Nothing. The events of my life to date had paled in comparison to that one selfless act of love that granted me eternal life regardless of my own inadequacies.

Jesus did this for me so that when the doctor called to tell me, "You have cancer," I could quote Psalm 118:17–18: "I shall not die, but live, and declare the works of the Lord. The Lord has chastened me severely, but he has not given me over to death."

Why would God give up such a priceless gift and make this ultimate sacrifice? The only feasible answer that my human brain can decipher is a deep, profound, and unadulterated love for an undeserving mankind. Never on my craziest day would I even think of sacrificing one hair on my own child's head to save anyone on the planet, much less an ungrateful stranger.

John 3:16–17 says: "For God so loved the world that He gave His only begotten Son, that whoever believes in Him should not perish but have everlasting life. For God did not send His Son into the world to condemn the world, but that the world through Him might be saved."

The owner of the cattle on a thousand hills gave his perfect and only son so that, when I got cancer, I would have a shot at healing, at redemption, and at eternal life. If God could give that much, how could I possibly ask him why I was sick?

The Perfect Storm

It's funny how a little bump in the road or break in the normal routine of our lives can throw us to our knees. I sometimes wonder if God allows us to have problems because he doesn't hear from us often enough. I was going way over my number of allotted cell phone minutes to God and was glad he wasn't cutting off my service. I wanted him to hear from me all day, every day.

Not only did I pray non-stop, but I made certain that Satan knew exactly where I stood and that I was not afraid of him (1 Thessalonians 5:17–18).

I was blessed and highly favored. I would not live in fear. I would not cower to the principalities of darkness (Ephesians 6:12). I would not succumb to Satan's plan for my life. I did not know what tomorrow would hold for me, but I certainly knew who held tomorrow (Matthew 6:33–34).

One afternoon in my living room, when Satan was trying to tell me that I wasn't going to be around much longer, I let him know just what I thought. Again, I always like to keep it real so there is no miscommunication. I was in an empty living room, shouting at the top of my lungs.

"You cannot defeat me. You do not win. You cannot destroy me or my home. You cannot take a mother away from her children or a wife away from her husband. You cannot beat me. I am a winner. I am a victor. I am bigger and better than you could ever hope to be. I am a child of the living God. The royal blood of heaven flows through my veins. Heaven doesn't even like you; that's why you got booted out. But that's where I'm going one day, and it won't be anytime soon. You do not have the power to take my life. You didn't give me life. You don't control my life. You cannot affect how I react in any given situation. You do not own me. I was purchased with precious blood. You can give it your very best shot, but if all you have is a little cancer to throw my way, then you suck! Bring it on!"

The next day my husband graciously drove me to the store and placed my purse in the space behind my car seat without my knowledge. I'm sure he felt like *Driving Miss Daisy*, but he never complained about any of it. Since I was still in a lot of pain from the surgery, I was ready to crutch my way over to the store scooter, get my groceries, and get out as quickly as possible. Normally I would peruse every aisle, but I was in no mood to hang out, much to my husband's delight.

As Jim paid for the groceries, I slowly inched my way through the parking lot to my Suburban. The Texas humidity was in full force, and I was sweating from the energy I had exerted by dragging my enormous leg just a few feet. I was overjoyed at the thought of an air conditioned ride home, as Jim quickly caught up to my hampered gait with the grocery basket.

Before I heard the familiar beep of the key fob, I reached for my car door and noticed that it was unlocked. I assumed my husband was too busy hoisting me out of the car to remember to lock up when an ominous feeling struck us both in the same instant. My mouth went dry. The door to my Suburban had been jimmied with a screw driver and the lock had been completely destroyed.

My husband thought I left my purse in the car on purpose; now it was gone, along with several other items in my car. I was steaming. Satan had gone too far, and it was becoming increasingly obvious that he was not going to give me a break.

Over the next few months our home computer crashed, our clothes washer and dryer died, our dishwasher burned up, our microwave exploded and caught on fire, our small appliances broke, my husband's tires blew out on his truck, and every TV in our house stopped working without explanation. We could have started our own game show "What Will Break Next?"

Satan was unrelenting in his pursuit, and each round made me more determined to fight that much harder. I learned a great deal about perseverance through these explosions and continued to remind Satan on a daily basis what a complete moron he was. I was not giving up that easily.

I began to read Psalm 62:11–12, which says, "…That power belongs to God. Also to You, O Lord, belongs mercy; For You render to each one according to his work." Satan was not going to deter me from my ultimate goal of total healing. He could destroy my possessions, but he didn't have the power to destroy me. I had cancer, but cancer would *never* have me.

It was June 20, 2006, my brother Chris's birthday. Dr.

Colbert, a dear friend and fantastic doctor from Florida, told me that he once had a patient with leiomyosarcoma. Not only was it very rare, but it was also extremely aggressive. He advised me to get to a sarcoma oncologist "yesterday."

By this time the news was spreading like wildfire as more of our friends and church members found out about my diagnosis. As a family, we had gathered very few facts on my condition. There was no consenting professional opinion. We did not know how long the cancer had been in my body or how far it had spread, how severe or aggressive it was, what stage, how long I was supposed to live, or what the first step would be for my treatment if any was available to me.

I knew that M.D. Anderson would be treating me, and that was the extent of my sarcoma knowledge. Having not been tested by a specialist, I had no idea what I was truly facing. I only knew that time would tell but didn't know if time was on my side.

The rumors that were spreading were anything but good. "Did you hear that Tish has cancer? It's really bad; I think she's going to die." And these were the Christians. These were the precious soldiers who were calling and asking if the doctors would be amputating my leg or if my very young children understood that I might be dying. *Who in their right mind would tell a toddler their mother was dying?*

My email was filling at an alarming rate with tales of woe from people who had lost loved ones to cancer and held out little hope for me. Others had already walked a mile in my shoes and offered encouragement; they were a breath of fresh air. Still, the "Negative Nellies" were coming out in droves and multiplying by the minute. It was as if they wanted me to call and make my funeral arrangements while I still had the energy to dial the phone.

Several felt obligated to tell me they had experience with this type of cancer and knew of people dying within ninety days of their diagnosis. Some wanted to "share" with me that even though they were sure the cancer would take my life, they would continue praying for my family. Most wanted to know how many of my body parts would be chopped off.

One college friend called to swap stories about what a drag it was to walk around on crutches all day. Right about the time I was about to ask him if he was even serious about comparing his skiing accident to my cancer, I realized it was time to take action. Enough was enough. Satan had overplayed his hand, and it was time to kick him back to the curb and remind him that he could not steal my joy (James 1:2–4).

I put out a very brief but succinct email to everyone I could think of, letting them know the very small bit of data we had on sarcomas. This quick note explained that I would soon be headed to the number one hospital in the world for my particular brand of cancer, with the number one sarcoma specialist, and expected nothing but the best results. At this point I made it very clear that my family was thanking God for my complete healing, which was already on the way (Psalm 63:3–5). We knew God could and would heal me; we just didn't know how or when.

My email continued with a definitive plan of how I wanted people to pray for me. If they did not believe I could be healed and agree to start thanking God for my total healing, I asked them to please not lift me up in prayer at all. I did not want people praying for me who did not have faith that God in his mercy could reach out his arm and absolutely heal me beyond a shadow of a doubt. I didn't want people praying for me who were asking for my healing after my leg was amputated. I wanted to remain whole.

I know that God's perfect healing and sometimes his answer is death. In my case, I wanted to enlist not-so-secret agents here on earth to petition the heavenlies for my total and complete healing so that I could continue being a wife and mother, sister and aunt, friend and co-worker. I wanted prayer warriors with worn-out kneepads and well-used Bibles that weren't afraid to step up to the plate and lay it on the line. I wanted people praying for me who knew God personally and had a relationship with him; those who understood what a prayer closet is.

In the Bible, Matthew uses the Lord's Prayer as the ultimate example of how to pray (Matthew 6:7–8). Pray specifically. My dad always says, "When you pray, don't pray for a bicycle. Pray for the red Schwinn bicycle from Sears, so that when you receive it, you know it was from God."

I did not want to pass go or collect two hundred dollars. I was focused on the prize and heading right to the finish line with my track shoes on. I'm not much of a game player, and I wasn't going to use this as an opportunity to start. It was time to get on my face before the Lord and tell him in no uncertain terms that I wanted to *live*.

I was about to turn into David fighting Goliath (Psalm 18:1–6). So I told Satan, "I come to you in the name of the Lord. Consider yourself defeated *again*." And I picked up my sling shot and started to swing.

Satan could break my washing machine, but he could

not break my spirit. Though I was smack dab in the center of the weakest moment of my life, I knew that in my weakness he is strong. And if God is for me, who could be against me (Psalm 27)?

The out-of-control rumor mill came to an abrupt halt as my email was forwarded to hundreds of people all over the world. My attempt to keep my cancer diagnosis under wraps until I had a more definitive picture had become a complete and utter failure, but finally we were all praying for the same thing—total healing. It was time to enjoy a few short days before leaving for my initiation to M.D. Anderson.

One afternoon I visited my daughter's kindergarten class at school in my wheelchair. My leg was still recovering from having the tumor removed, and crutches were only an option when I had a very short distance to travel. I was hoping the wheelchair wouldn't scare my daughter's friends and cause her any undue concern. She was used to my "bad" leg, but her friends were not. You just never know what will run through the mind of a child, and I prayed that the wheelchair wouldn't cause any major crisis.

These thoughts were in the forefront of my mind when one of the little boys in the class came up and, with a huge smile on his face, told me, "Mckenzie's Mom, we have all been praying for you in our class very hard, even our teacher." It was all I could do to choke back the tears as this tiny person looked up at me without fear or reservation but with total confidence that everything was going to be all right. It was an instant lesson that spoke volumes to me.

That afternoon the class sent a get-well card home for me in my daughter's folder. It brought me to tears as I remembered the sweet words of the little boy and thought about the wonderful innocence of children. The Bible says that little children would lead them. Here were these precious tiny people who were willing to pray for my healing, even though they didn't remotely understand what was going on. They were willing to pray with total faith, believing that I would absolutely receive healing. Why was it so easy for these small children to understand basic Bible principals and pray without a shred of doubt when the adults surrounding them did nothing but complicate the picture?

I was grateful my daughter attended a Christian school where she was allowed to pray, and even more grateful that she was too young to understand exactly why she was praying (Proverbs 22:6). The web of favor that was shrouding my children from the truth was an endless source of comfort to me, as it was difficult to breathe when I imagined what their lives would be like without me. When things seemed like they were too good to be true, and my family was shielded from unspeakable horrors, all I could say was, *"But God."*

The cards that came from the school were just the beginning. I began to receive emails from people I didn't know in places I didn't know existed. Preachers, bishops, rabbis, military personnel, government agents, janitors, cafeteria workers, teachers, daycare workers, bankers, governors, powerful businessmen, women, and even children began to email and send cards. Governors and senators were praying for me, along with priests and rabbis. It seemed that my support system was growing by leaps and bounds, in ways I had never before imagined.

As thousands of emails started pouring in from just about everywhere, I began to discover a new theme in the snowstorm of emails that hit my "inbox" faster than I could respond. It was an overwhelming relief with a resounding positive note that tugged at my heartstrings and made me understand that this cancer was bringing me closer to my divine destiny. Did I think God gave me the cancer? No. But I knew this cancer did not surprise God and prayed that it would be used to help others.

What shocked me and caught me completely by surprise was how God used the cancer to help and change *me* for the better. This new and seemingly endless stream of emails typically sounded something like this: "You don't know me, but your dad prayed for my cancer in 1980. I'm still here, and now my family is praying for you." "We have listened to your dad preach for the past thirty-five years, and we want you to know that we are praying for you every day as a family." "Your mom told us about your situation, and we are praying for you in Africa."

Cancer survivors started coming out of the woodwork to encourage me. This was a complete 360 from some of the previous emails I had been receiving and a most welcome change. The relief that swept over me like a cleansing tidal wave was an emotional farewell to the negativity that had once tried to overtake my life. If others had lived to tell about it, I could too. A profound sense of relief swept through the recesses of my mind, as I now only had to deal with the reality of my cancer, not speculation and rumor.

Still, I could not get over the sheer number of total strangers who wanted to pray and stand in the gap for me, who made a daily commitment to petition the Lord on my behalf. It would have been so easy to walk away from a complete stranger, yet they wanted to go out of their way to let me know they were praying for me in every state in the union and in foreign places I had never seen. They were strangers to me, but not to God, and that was what mattered.

It is not at all unusual for complete strangers to approach me and call me by name. Many times they have seen me at church or watch my dad on TV, and occasionally they have attended school with one of my siblings or attended a conference with my mother. So when a blonde lady I had never met before approached me in the middle of my neighborhood Target, I thought nothing of it.

She said, "You don't know me, but God told me to stop here and talk to you." She had my attention. Normally when people tell me, "You don't know me," it is followed by them calling me by name and saying, "I have known you since you were this big," as they hold their hand at their knee cap. But this obvious stranger hadn't given any of the usual responses, which further intrigued me.

I knew the woman standing in front of me was either a total nut case having a manic moment, or this was absolute divine intervention in my life. I was looking for the store security guard just in case, and holding on tightly to my new purse.

She looked me straight in the eye and said, "I want you to know that you are totally healed. The Lion of Judah is roaring for you, and when the Lion of Judah speaks, *everyone* listens. I should not be here this morning, but God told me to come to this Target, completely out of my way, and talk to the first lady that came up on my right. I am late for work, but I felt this word was too important not to deliver. I don't know you or your situation, but whatever you are going through, you must know that God is on your side." And with that, she turned on her heels and went right out into the parking lot.

You could have knocked me over with a feather as cold chills began to spiral through my body. God had sent a total stranger to find me and deliver a healing message at Target (Matthew 28:20). I wasn't in church or at a prayer meeting. I was at Target! God had sent his messenger to find me right where I was. I didn't know whether to laugh or cry as I stood there in total shock, staring into space. My feet were made of stone, and I couldn't move in any direction as the joy of the Lord flooded my soul (Psalm 67).

That morning gave whole new meaning to shopping being a religious experience. No specialist had even defined the scope of my illness, much less confirmed my healing; yet God used a total stranger to reiterate that he was totally in control. God had shown up, completely unexpected, and let me know that he was going to be the fourth man in my fire. In case I wasn't listening when my friends and family told me, he grabbed an extra stranger off the highway to swing by Target and run the message by me one more time.

Unrelenting Grace

God was weaving a circle of strong prayer warriors to cover me during my greatest hour of need. An hour that at times seemed like an eternity. I was continually amazed by his mercy and touched to the core by the sheer number of people who continued to keep up with my progress on a weekly basis. These people were genuinely concerned with my well being as if I was their own beloved family member. They didn't ask about my condition once and then continue on with their own lives. They kept up with my progress from start to finish (Galatians 6:2).

The support system that began to cocoon itself around me seemed like an impenetrable barrier that guarded me from the anxiety and fear that normally goes hand-in-hand with a cancer diagnosis (Psalm 23:4). I wasn't pretending to not be afraid and putting on a brave face; I was genuinely not afraid. And since I am normally a person who holds a Ph.D. in worry, this was a new position of power for me that I deeply treasured.

I continued to receive daily emails of encouragement that

were often accompanied by beautiful flowers and thoughtful gifts. One that really touched me came from my former professors at the University of the Incarnate Word in San Antonio. These precious ladies sent a soft pink baby blanket and a beautiful rosary they made by hand especially for me. This arrived with a sweet letter stating that they were praying for me every day and fully expecting God's best.

I was instructed to take the blanket with me to any treatments or to use it any time I needed to be reminded I was covered in prayer. I was instructed to pass the blanket on to someone else in need when I was healed.

The gifts that arrived at my door or at the church on my behalf were astonishingly thoughtful and exceptionally kind. With each personal outpouring of kindness, I became increasingly insulated against the harsh reality of my current existence and more deeply enveloped in the warmth of God's love. I was entangled in a web of comfort and support.

Rabbi Scheinberg, a dear friend of my father's, called to tell me he had been praying for me in Jerusalem at the Wailing Wall. His congregation was praying for me daily at the temple in San Antonio as well. Rabbi has a very warm and kind voice, and he chooses his words deliberately. He called to tell me, "Tish, we are praying for you in stereo." His kindness touched the very center of my heart, as there were no words to express my appreciation for his prayers and the prayers of his congregation. I was being lifted before Jehovah God by both Christians and Jews alike.

While Rabbi was praying for me at the Wailing Wall, another group of our friends from Colorado (who did not know Rabbi), the Morrisons, ran into him there. When the Morrisons explained they were praying for a girl in Texas who had cancer, they all realized they were praying for the same person—me. God had taken groups of people around the world to lift me up in a country that he considers the apple of his eye.

The magnitude of what was happening hit me like a bolt of lightning. God began to tell me this was not at all about me but was totally about him. This was his hour to shine, his time to show off. He had the attention of people all over San Antonio and various parts of the world. Like cancer, God is no respecter of persons. These people from all walks of life, various denominations, and across every socioeconomic bracket were "praying for me in stereo," and I found great comfort in that (Psalm 103:1–3).

I felt like Daniel in the lion's den with impending danger on every side. I was down but not out. What was meant for evil, God was using for his good (Genesis 50:20). I had complete faith that he would deliver me.

It was very hard for me to be silent, or to sit and wait, but what were my options here? I could choose to trust in the Lord with all my heart and lean not on my own understanding, or live in fear (Proverbs 3:5–8). Not a lot of choices.

I didn't know how my cancer could be news to anyone else. I didn't personally know that many people, but evidently a lot of people knew about me. One person turned into ten, ten turned into a hundred, then a thousand and then tens of thousands. People began calling and writing from all over the globe.

God's total peace wrapped around me like a warm cashmere blanket in the dead of winter.

I had done nothing to deserve this measure of grace and was only beginning to understand the depth of his love for me. God's mercies were raining down like a torrential thunderstorm. As one African Bishop wrote, "The name of your cancer is leiomyosarcoma, but we know the name that is above all other names." This name would be my salvation (Philippians 2:9–11).

Cancer came into my life in the blink of an eye, like a thief breaking into a home at mid-day, taking an unsuspecting family hostage. There was no rhyme or reason. I had not done anything to ask for this or to cause this physical reaction in my body. It was simply one of those life experiences that you have no control over. Regardless of the bleak forecast, I made it a priority to give thanks for the blessings surrounding my current circumstances. I knew I was in the right place at the right time, so I continued relishing the goodness of God's favor in the valley of the shadow of death (Psalm 27).

In my pre-diagnosis life, I was a good person, but I wasn't doing all that I could. I was in constant motion, helping many great causes, but not truly reaching for my divine destiny like I should have been. I had become complacent and lax in many areas, choosing to relax when I should have done more. I began to crave pleasing God in every aspect of my life, knowing that one day I would be judged not only for what I did, but also for what I did not do. God very succinctly began stripping me of those things that were unnecessarily important in my life.

The first thing to go was my beloved shoes. I never met a pair of heels I didn't like. The higher the heel, the bigger the platform, the funkier the shoe, the flashier, the better. After my initial surgery I couldn't even wear shoes because my foot was so swollen. Heels were out of the question. I was limited to "fashionable" house shoes and, once in a while, some hot pink Crocs. My once limitless shoe collection had dwindled down to a few simple choices that I could barely squeeze onto my fat right foot. These choices were also trendy among nursing home dwellers, so I wasn't exactly thrilled with my current selection.

A tremendous amount of healing took place before I was promoted from fluffy leopard slippers to trendy slip-on tennis shoes. (I hadn't owned tennis shoes in over a decade because tennis shoes are for runners, and I have had no desire to run since about the age of five). Previously I had believed that tennis shoes and ballet flats were for old ladies who wore support hose, but they were quickly becoming a fan favorite in my empty closet.

I began to painstakingly give my very popular size eight shoes away to women who needed them but couldn't afford them. They were beautiful, expensive, designer shoes in every shape and color. I didn't need them to define myself or what I was about. I wanted someone else to get good wear out of them, because my life was taking a major turn after being thrown a curve ball. It was time to start peeling the proverbial layers of the onion.

I wanted to make myself over from the inside out so that every second I had left would count for something that actually mattered. Who needs to be remembered for a fantastic shoe collection? I would leave that to Imelda Marcos. I wanted to make a *real* difference in the lives of others, not just give out fashion tips.

My husband was shocked to see me getting rid of so many

boxes of shoes, as I only owned one pair of flats that I saved in the back of my closet for a rainy day in a total act of fashion desperation. My rainy day had come, and it was time to move forward to the destination that God had in mind for me.

The Healing Balm of a Psalm

Hear my cry, O God; attend to my prayer. From the end of the earth I will cry to you, when my heart is overwhelmed; lead me to the rock that is higher than I. For you have been a shelter for me, a strong tower from the enemy. I will abide in your tabernacle forever; I will trust in the shelter of your wings. Selah. For you, O God, have heard my vows; you have given *me* the heritage of those who fear your name. You will prolong the king's life, his years as many generations. He shall abide before God forever. Oh, prepare mercy and truth, which may preserve him! So I will sing praise to your name forever, that I may daily perform my vows.

Psalm 61

He who dwells in the secret place of the Most High shall abide under the shadow of the Almighty. I will say of the Lord, "He is my refuge and my fortress; my God, in him I will trust." Surely he shall deliver you from the snare of the fowler and from the perilous pestilence. He shall cover you with his feathers, and under his wings you shall take refuge; his truth shall be your shield and buckler. You shall not be afraid of the terror by night, nor of the arrow that flies by day, nor of the pestilence that walks in darkness, nor of the destruction that lays waste at noonday. A thousand may fall at your side, and ten thousand at your right hand; but it shall not come near you. Only with your eyes shall you look, and see the reward of the wicked. Because you have made the Lord, who is my refuge, even the Most High, your dwelling place, no evil shall befall you, nor shall any plague come near your dwelling; for he shall give his angels charge over you, to keep you in all your ways. In their hands they shall bear you up, lest you dash your foot against a stone. You shall tread upon the lion and the cobra, the young lion and the serpent you shall trample underfoot. Because he has set his love upon me, therefore I will deliver him; I will set him on high, because he has known my name. He shall call upon me, and I will answer him; I will be with him in trouble; I will deliver him and honor him. With long life I will satisfy him, and show him my salvation.

Psalm 91

Psalm 61 was the scripture God gave me. My heart was most certainly overwhelmed at every turn. Some days I was over-whelmed by God's mercy and grace. Some days I felt too young to be headed for life in a cancer ward. And still other days I was just plain physically exhausted. Many days I was astonished by the kindness of those around me who were constantly willing to lend a helping hand at every turn, just out of sheer generosity and pure love.

I was not overwhelmed like a bride is on her wedding day, or during the many days that lead up to the ceremony as plans are feverishly made, while budgets run low and tension runs high. I was not overwhelmed like a new parent who is so sleep-deprived they are wondering if they will be the first person to die from lack of rest and proper nutrition.

I was overwhelmed like someone who had no idea what the next moment of her life would entail, if she would ever return to any state of normalcy again, if her next set of doctor's visits would render good news, or if her family would be forced to live without her after a nice potluck reception. I was overwhelmed, and at the same time, I was completely at peace.

Psalm 91 was the scripture my dad's mom, Grandma Hagee, had read when she was fighting cancer in the '80s. Since I was thirty years younger than she was when I was diagnosed, Psalm 61 somehow seemed fitting. I read both scriptures every day. I memorized them for the days when my head throbbed and my eyes burned so badly that it hurt to crack them open.

I lived in the Psalms and thrived in the healing balm that they provided for my soul. They made my heart sing on days when it felt like breaking from sheer exhaustion. The Psalms helped me maintain a definitive mental picture of my overall goal.

Psalm 61 especially hit home with me because I had been given a rich, Christian heritage and had taken it all for granted. I could recite parts of familiar sermons or old jokes, anecdotes and sermon illustrations, and I took it all for granted. I knew I would be sitting in the same pew, listening to my dad preach until his last breath came out of his lungs with one foot still in the pulpit and one hand on the microphone. On a slow day, my dad has more energy and accomplishes more than I do in a busy week. The thought of my dad burying me had never remotely crossed my mind.

During any given church service I would think about what I needed to do later in the week: make my grocery list, think about loans at work that needed to close, and scribble notes of errands I needed to run or places I needed to take my children. I paid attention about half of the time when I wasn't making mental notes of who was in attendance. I had been in the audience of one of the country's greatest Bible preachers for almost four decades and had taken those years of teaching for granted.

I was very blessed indeed, and I would not take it for granted again. I asked God to forgive me and to start directing my path for this very special time in my life.

I wanted the doors that needed to be opened in my life to be thrown open with ease and the doors that needed to be closed to be sealed shut. The podiatrist who had initially excised the tumor from my leg recommended a doctor that couldn't see me for several weeks due to personal vacation plans. I knew this was not our guy, as the only real fact I knew about my sarcoma was that it grew very quickly. That door was closed.

One of our family doctors, Dr. Schnitzler, recommended Dr. Kalter, an oncologist at the Cancer Therapy and Research Center in San Antonio, for an immediate secondary consult. I was going to M.D. Anderson for treatment as soon as I could get in, but I wanted to see an oncologist as soon as possible to find out more about leiomyosarcoma and how to treat it.

I wanted to talk to a specialist and get some insight on what might be in store for me, and to ask if anyone had ever survived this type of cancer before. Though the black, hazy fog and numbness were gone, the constant ebb and flow of questions swimming around in my brain had only increased in intensity since my diagnosis. I wanted a doctor with some expertise on the topic at hand to give me one shred of medical hope. I knew specific details could only come from a sarcoma specialist, but I decided to give a non-sarcoma oncologist with *only* forty-plus years of experience a shot at giving me his opinion.

Dr. Kalter was the sweetest doctor you ever want to meet. He was very kind and expressed genuine concern when he examined my hideously swollen and bruised leg, which had far surpassed the purple and green cactus stage at this point. I told him that originally two doctors had tried on separate occasions to drain what they believed to be a ganglion cyst. Dr. Kalter was concerned that the needle tracks might have spread the cancer cells through my blood system and into other parts of my body.

Fantastic! The hits just kept coming. And what do we have behind curtain number two, Bob? Another potential life-threatening problem.

In case I didn't have enough questions after my original diagnosis, the fact that I was just made aware that the cancer could have been spread unknowingly to my blood stream sent me into overdrive. Surely someone was going to pop into my examination room and tell me I had just been Punk'd. But there was no Ashton Kutcher in sight, only Dr. Kalter.

I was happy to see an oncologist with a smile on his face that reached up to his sparkling eyes. In the span of a few short days, I had gone from delivering meals to friends after their own hospital visits to becoming a regular fixture on the hospital scene. I had a book in my purse, prepared for the inevitable long wait in the lobby that was laminated with out-of-date magazines, and was no longer impatient when the doctors took up my time with the same set of questions I could now recite in two languages in my sleep. It was just a part of the journey.

Dr. Kalter had trained at M.D. Anderson, and graciously volunteered to help me with any part of my treatment or recovery after my visit to Houston. He was the first oncologist I consulted with and was a true breath of fresh air.

Two days later, Red McCombs, a local San Antonio businessman and former owner of the Minnesota Vikings, made a phone call to M.D. Anderson on my behalf. On June 26, 2006, I was on my way to my first appointment at the largest medical center in the United States. It had only been seven days since my diagnosis, but it felt like a lifetime had passed since I had received that fated call, instantly and irrevocably changing the course of my life.

The Mecca That is
M.D. Anderson

As Diana and I were driving to Houston for the very first time, she was conducting business on the phone as usual, and I was leisurely flipping through the pages of the latest gossip magazine. The trip from San Antonio to Houston takes about three hours, so we had plenty of time to burn. What better way to waste time than by reading about what's going on in Hollywood?

I was lost in my magazine when Diana hung up her phone and looked directly at me (and yes, she was still driving). "I want you to please forgive me for anything that I have ever done to offend you. At a time like this, you need to get everything in your life in order and make sure you have forgiven everyone for whatever they may have done to you."

Whoa! The magnitude of the sincerity in her request sliced through the mindless banter I had just been reading, and I in turn asked her to forgive me for anything I had done.

Diana has been my step-mother since I was six years old. I cannot consciously remember a time when she was not a part of my life. Sometimes I can't remember what I ate for dinner last night or my next door neighbor's name. Here she was asking me to forgive her for decades worth of offenses. Just when I started to prepare for a very long ride naming past offenses, she shrugged her shoulders and said it had already rolled off her back.

As Diana picked up the phone to make another call, I started thinking about God. How much had he let roll off his back? How many times had I offended him or let him down? How many times had he requested that I do something, and I turned the other way? Could I have reached out to more people, helped more in distress?

I knew it was a very real possibility that I could be standing in front of the Son of God in very short order, and I wanted him to forgive me for all of those missed opportunities, things I should have or could have done but instead decided to go to the movies. I wanted the opportunity to make it right but knew that opportunity might never come.

My mind was the quintessential man vs. man struggle. On the one hand I knew that God was going to heal me, but on the other hand I didn't know how or when. I also knew that the method of healing was up to God. Would I lose my leg before my healing came? Would my perfect healing mean that my body would only be made whole in death? Would I have to teach my children that death is a part of life as they were starting elementary school? I only knew that I had to make each day count for something while remaining focused on my goal of defeating the enemy that had temporarily claimed my body.

As we motored up the road, I used the remainder of the

ride to thank God for his blessings and recount the great things that were happening in my life. I never finished the magazine, and by the time I looked up, we were at the hotel. I was elated, as I was ready to run to my room and fall into bed, clothes and all.

I quickly began to rifle through my bags in search of a toothbrush when my mind inconveniently started a virtual tug of war with fear and doubt. The reality of impending death set in, and I began to experience true, bone-chilling, paralyzing fear for the very first time. Now that I was finally in Houston, I was just a few short days away from being handed a medical chart full of facts regarding my very near future. I would be given medical diagnoses to determine if I was going to have a future.

Thoughts of the endless ways cancer could ravage my body began flooding my senses as fear began to reign supreme and my mind wandered in a thousand morbid directions. Fear is an all-consuming emotion that can overpower your rational senses before you realize it. It can grip you like an invisible, choking hand and suffocate you in a matter of seconds.

Fear renders you powerless and systematically begins to control and destroy every aspect of your life. Fear is a manipulative tool that Satan uses to place himself in a position of power over us, to divide us from the Word of God (Hebrews 4:12). Of course, prayer trumps fear. Where prayer exists, fear cannot thrive.

The Bible has 365 different references that say "do not fear." Now I am no math genius, but I think that is one "do not fear" for each calendar day. If God can write "do not fear" that many times, I am pretty sure he does not want me to fear.

When I start to worry about what I can't control, I become full of fear and doubt. Stress begins to run my life, and I become reactive instead of proactive. Matthew 6:27 says, "Which of you by worrying can add one cubit to his stature?" A cubit is eighteen inches. Since I am only five feet two inches tall, this would make me eligible for the WNBA overnight. If I gained eighteen inches in height every time I worried about something, my body would wrap around the globe several times over.

Fear is always the first and biggest obstacle to overcome in any serious situation, but it can quickly develop into a fire-breathing dragon in a life-threatening situation. I was not going to allow fear to control me. If I gave in to fear and doubt, I could quickly be consumed by the cancer, propelled into overdrive by a high stress level.

However, not being afraid is easier said than done. Make no mistake. Satan loves to play mind games when doctors diagnose you with a terminal disease or you suddenly find your life taking a change for the worse when least expected.

Knowing all of these practical and well-recited tidbits on how fear can control a situation was not helping me one bit with my personal battle over fear in my comfy hotel room. I was in my own personal hell.

While I was mentally hammering out my plan of attack for my hospital visit in the morning, my leg began to throb like never before. Was I just imagining this, or was the fear increasing my pain level? It was 11:00 p.m., and my right leg was black and blue up to my knee. (After my surgery, the only area that was bruised was right around my ankle bone. At this point in the game, the swelling and discoloration had far surpassed these original borders to almost encompass my knee cap.) My foot had become so swollen that my toes looked like miniature sausages.

Even though my leg was hurting, I knew I would get an uninterrupted night of sleep, because there were no children in the hotel room to wake me up in the middle of the night to ask me for juice or help with a quick trip to the restroom. Lindsay Wagner and her Sleep Number Bed had nothing on me. Having shoved down a quick dinner from room service, I was ready to crash.

I fell into a deep slumber the second my head met the oversized down pillow, but not for long. The fear that had been taunting me in my room before dinner became an unwelcome guest in my dreams. I was being hunted, and Satan was doing his best to destroy me.

Satan began screaming in my head, *Your life is over. This cancer is a death sentence for you. Your husband lost his mother to cancer, and now he's going to lose you. You will not see another birthday for either of your children. They will grow up without a mother and will be in and out of counseling for the rest of their lives trying to understand how a loving God would take their mother from them at such a young age. Your husband will be forced to sell your home because he can't afford that house without your income. You can't work or help your family financially if you're dead. Your children won't be able to go to college. Your life is over and so is theirs.*

I woke up in a cold sweat with the deafening sound of my own heartbeat ringing loudly in my ears. I felt powerless against the raging sea of fear inside me. Very few things in life had ever scared me, but I was now meeting a new enemy I had not truly been confronted by before, raw and relentless fear.

Just hours before, I had been experiencing an all-time emotional and spiritual high in anticipation of finally receiving some concrete answers. Now I felt light years away from that safe lining of security. Physically my foot was throbbing unmercifully and felt like it would surely crack open at any given moment from the pressure building up inside. I could feel the constant pounding of each nerve ending in my brain. My entire body ached with fever and shook with chills as if I had the flu.

I knew I would need to go to the emergency room soon if I could not get some type of relief from the agony that was rapidly starting to travel from my leg up to my head where a migraine was quickly forming at the base of my skull. I began to slowly hobble over to the bathroom, reaching for the hot water handle on the tub to begin steaming out the aches and pains that were racking my body from top to bottom.

I would have used an ice pick to relieve the pressure in my head if one had been handy, just anything to relieve the pain. When I reached the faucet, not one drop of hot water came out. The water was ice cold. I went to the sink. No hot water. I couldn't believe it! We were at a four-star hotel with no hot water in the middle of the night. Perfect.

I was sitting in the middle of the bathroom floor completely incensed by the lack of hot water, which only made my head and leg throb with greater intensity. I was sure the pounding in my brain was loud enough to wake everyone in the hotel, but at that moment I just didn't care. I wanted some relief!

There was nothing I could do to alleviate the pain even for one brief moment, so I tried to look at the bright side and battle the fear through the pain. If I was in pain that meant I was still alive. I was still able to fight. The battle wasn't over by a long shot.

I started thanking God for my healing. *I don't know what the doctors are going to tell me tomorrow, but I know that you hold tomorrow in the palm of your hand. I don't know how much cancer I have or how far it has spread, but I know that if you watch over the tiny sparrows, then you will surely take care of me. When I was born, you knew this day would come. Thank you for not telling me until now. This was not a surprise for you. You solved this problem before I knew it existed. If I was the only one to ever have cancer in the history of the universe, you still would have died on the cross just for me. Because of the stripes on your back, I am healed. I thank you for my healing. I accept my healing, not because of anything I have done, and certainly not because I deserve it, but because of your mercy and your grace. Thank you for loving me enough to die in my place. And to the spirit of fear, I speak to you directly. You have no place in my life. You cannot touch me. You cannot harm me, and you certainly cannot kill me. I send you back to the depths of hell where you came from in the name of Jesus and tell you that you have absolutely no power over me. Amen.*

By this time I was crawling on my hands and knees back to bed, the pain intensifying with every slight movement of my body. The surgical bandages on my foot and leg were wrapped so tightly they felt as if my circulation was being cut off and at any point my bandages would explode in all directions, much like the Incredible Hulk's t-shirt when he gets angry. As I reached down to rip the bandage from my foot, I very clearly heard God tell me, "Don't touch a thing. I am healing you from the top of your head to the soles of your feet."

Instantly there was no pain in any part of my body. No fever. No chills. I had to pinch myself to make sure this was really happening because just a few seconds before, the pain was excruciating and unrelenting. The fear was gone just as quickly as it had come. Within sixty seconds I was sleeping like a baby.

A few hours later I awoke with a smile on my face and a sense of renewed purpose. My focus was back on the Word of God, exactly where it needed to be. "This is the day that the Lord has made and I will rejoice and be glad in it" (Psalm 118:24). I was pumped and ready to begin the day. No matter what the doctors at M.D. Anderson told me during the next grueling week of testing and probing, I knew I had already been promised complete healing. And since God never fails, I knew his promise would ring true in due season.

Promise. Problem. Provision. I knew I had a problem. I knew the promise for me was found in many verses throughout the Bible but especially in Psalm 61. Now I needed a miraculous, supernatural provision to continue living.

When Diana woke up, I told her with absolute certainty and a smile on my face, "This is going to be a good day." Before we left for M.D. Anderson to meet with the doctors for the very first time, we read Psalm 61 and Psalm 91. Diana prayed for God's favor, that the doctors would relay any news in a positive way no matter how grave the reality.

The line had been drawn in the sand, and I finally felt like my battle plan was taking flight.

I reminded myself that I had to stay focused on the promise God had given me no matter what I saw or heard, but in that instant I could never have imagined the vivid display that would forever carve itself into my memory during the course of that day.

We got dressed quickly and drove to M.D. Anderson.

Now, my mind is a very colorful place, and I had envisioned a hospital something like the one my girls were born in. I never imagined anything of this magnitude. It took my breath away as we began to drive up the long street that houses the many buildings encompassed by M.D. Anderson.

This was a medical metropolis like nothing I had seen before. There were eight enormous numbered buildings in a row that each housed ten to fifteen floors. Smaller treatment centers were on the outskirts of these buildings, with everything connected by walkways, breezeways, and sidewalks. A golf cart would drive you from one building to the next if you could not make the walk.

From what I could see out of my car window, there were endless miles to walk in between floors and buildings, and I only had one good, pain-free leg. Where were we supposed to go, and how was I supposed to get there? Should I drop bread crumbs so I could find my way back?

Since I am directionally dysfunctional, it is always stressful for me to find a new place. I knew it would take about five seconds to get lost inside this mammoth collection of buildings. And since I wasn't wearing my shiny red shoes, I couldn't click my heels together and say, "There's no place like home."

My anxiety level was mounting as I took in the visible feast surrounding this monstrous hospital. We drove up to the main entrance, which was like Disney World without the rides and smiles. People of all shapes, colors, and sizes were everywhere. There were rows and rows of people getting out of cars and valets coming to assist them in and out of wheel-chairs. Did all of these people have cancer?

I couldn't believe what my eyes were telling me. There were people missing arms, legs, eyes, and other major chunks of their bodies. The lucky ones were only missing hair. Many couldn't walk. Most seemed to be carrying the weight of the world on their shoulders. Few were smiling.

Hundreds of wheelchairs were stacked in neat rows by the front door. The endless sea of people flooding the buildings was astonishing and instantly made me sick to my stomach. It was sensory overload. Surely I did not belong at this hospital with all of these sick people!

As the valet came to open my door and assist me into my wheelchair, I realized that I would indeed fit right in. As I rolled into the building, I looked around and saw the dense sea of cancer patients surrounding me at every angle. They were like ants scurrying everywhere. The patients were so prolific that they seemed to be dripping from the ceilings. Some were coming, some were going, some eating, some reading, and many were waiting. People were congregated in every section of the hospital and spilling over into the lob-bies. There were no empty waiting rooms or areas vacant of human suffering.

As I continued my visual digestion of my new surroundings, it hit me like a great sadness after an all-consuming personal loss. This hospital only services people who are dying. There are no new, healthy lives being brought into the world in this vast facility. My chipper attitude sunk like a lead balloon.

The patrons surrounding me as my wheelchair rolled by were more like me in that exact moment than I cared to admit. The startling reality of a cancer ward is shocking at best. This is not a vacation spot. No one chooses to visit here, but those who come understand. They know that health should never be taken for granted and that life is precious. If there was never any sickness or disease, how would we know that the gift of a healthy life is so priceless?

My mind was rapidly absorbing and sifting through the horrendous sights burning my eyes and becoming engrained in my memory bank. My brain was scanning too many ghastly sites to truly absorb and trying to keep up with the intensity of the horror show being played out before my very eyes. I was on a twisted carnival ride with no off button.

While approaching the hospital in the safety of my car, this place appeared to be an enormous Disney Land, filled with patrons shifting in and out of every possible square inch of the property. Once I was given a ticket to ride, this theme park took on a morbid tone that was much scarier than any Steven King novel. The room began to spin around me as the sights and sounds blurred together into one giant hum of frenzied activity.

I was ready to go home and check the box for some other treatment option. Surely I could go to a hospital full of well people with glowing skin who were sitting around laughing in the lobby and showing each other pictures of their children and grandchildren who still had all of their limbs intact, unlike the ones paraded before me now. I knew I had to stay, but I didn't want to turn into the girl next to me who was missing her leg or the kid on the other side with no eye and a bad attitude.

My hair could always grow back, and I could wear a different colored wig every day of the week, but I wanted to be healthy again. I wanted to talk about something besides cancer and spend time with the doctors that were my friends and not my diagnosticians. However, I had not lost my grasp on the stark reality I was facing which was becoming clearer as the seconds ticked by and the patients in front of me continued to enact a macabre play for an audience of one. Knowing I wanted a happy ending to my own story, I decided right there to pull myself up by the bootstraps and prepare for my first official round of cancer tests.

Diana was pushing my wheelchair as we entered the ice cold lobby, which was a welcome break from the Houston humidity. My heart broke for her. Here she was, pushing me into the very same hospital where her sister, Rosie, was treated more than thirty-two years ago at a time when chemo was the latest and most innovative treatment.

Rosie lost her four-year battle with neomyosarcoma at the age of eighteen. I couldn't imagine the agony Diana must be enduring with each step, while memories of her sister flooded her mind. I greatly admired the amount of courage it must have taken for her to come with me, and I was grateful to be with someone who sadly had too much experience with a disease I was just now truly learning about on an all-too-personal level.

Upon entering the main building we were greeted by Cyn, my personal patient advocate, who extended a warm greeting on behalf of the hospital. Immediately my anxiety about finding the right room for my appointment was relieved. I wouldn't need those bread crumbs after all, since she would be following my case as long as I was treated at M.D. Anderson. After handing us her card, Cyn led the way to the business office where I was to register as an official patient. By this time I was a pro at filling out hospital paperwork and assumed this would be more of the same.

Wrong! I was completely thrown for a loop when the hospital administrative assistant asked me if I wanted to request a DNR (do not resuscitate) order. When I explained that I was just here for a consult and some testing, she said, "Yes, and during your treatment here, if something should happen, do you want us to resuscitate you?" That was certainly a question I hadn't been asked during any of my previous hospital stays.

When the assistant looked at me, I could tell she wasn't expecting a, "We'll cross that bridge when we come to it" type of answer. I was just here today to find out more about the type of cancer I had and any type of possible treatments. I wasn't coming here to die and certainly hadn't planned on needing resuscitation before the week ended.

I could feel my skin turning a deeper shade of lily white. Was she serious? I didn't even feel sick other than the sudden nausea that hit me with this new line of questioning.

Just when I thought the water was safe to swim again, Jaws showed up and stuck her fin out in the water.

"Do you have a living will? If not, we can help you put one together."

A living will? Maybe she didn't see my birth date. I wasn't even halfway to retirement yet. I was still trying to decide what I really wanted to be when I grew up. Last week I was diagnosed with cancer; I was finally getting my arms around the *c* word being attached to my name, and this total stranger wanted to know if I had a living will. I was afraid to ask what would come next. Check, please.

With my blood pressure at an all-time high and the paperwork behind us, Cyn escorted us to the tenth floor, where I was introduced to the M.D. Anderson Sarcoma Center. I had no idea what to expect, but prepared myself for more of what the lobby had to offer. A quick scan of the waiting area confirmed more missing limbs and broken hearts. It was as if I had walked into the middle of a war zone and could not find my way to the DMZ (demilitarized zone).

I never wanted to be a part of *this* crowd. I never wanted to be a part of *any* crowd, to just complacently fit in. I liked being my own person, having my own personality and style. I never concerned myself with what those around me thought about my fashion sense, my hair cut or color, as long as I knew I was living according to God's Word. It's okay to be different. I was happy to be me.

As I looked around the waiting room, I replayed that fated phone call from the doctor in my head that I had now heard a million times. "You have leiomyosarcoma." I no longer wanted to be different. I wanted to have the same kind of cancer as everyone else. I wanted to have the kind of cancer that was common and easy to fix. I didn't want to stand out in the cancer crowd or be a part of a clique that rarely smiled or laughed.

More than that I wanted someone to tell me about a great new piece of technology that had just been discovered because I was the ninety-ninth person that day with the same problem. But here I was, feeling like the Lone Ranger. I was the only one I knew who had ever been diagnosed with this type of cancer, and as the song goes, "One is the loneliest number."

My life to date had not been a cake walk, but nothing had prepared me for the gut-wrenching reality I was now facing. I could literally be wasting away while I was sitting in the waiting room.

I started to take a closer look at my surroundings and found huge pictures of people plastered all over the walls throughout every hallway in the Sarcoma Center. Who were these people? I had plenty of time on my hands before they would inevitably call my name, so I started wandering around. Each picture showed a cancer survivor, usually enjoying their favorite hobby. A written caption underneath each smiling face briefly stated the type of cancer they had conquered and punctuated the fact that a positive attitude helped them stay alive.

Between the picture and the description was the type of cancer they had with a huge red line through it. They had won! They had defeated the cancer and wanted to tell others their story. Staring into the eyes of these photographed survivors was an amazing source of encouragement for a new patient like me.

It was, in fact, a former M.D. Anderson patient who made these lovely displays. She came to the hospital as a teenage girl, asking her sarcoma oncologist if anyone ever survived what she had. He said, "Of course." To prove it to her, he gave her the names and numbers of survivors to contact for support.

After her treatments, she was so grateful that she went to nursing school and became his nurse. She had taken these "survivor" pictures to give others hope. From what I could see, they were working. The pictures and stories were incredibly uplifting.

My name was finally called, and Diana and I followed the nurse into the examination room, our frayed emotions on our sleeves. Lindsey was the first oncological nurse I met at M.D. Anderson. She was exceptionally kind, and her positive attitude just oozed out of every pore in her body. She was upbeat and friendly, but most of all she was real. I was more than ready to see a face that held a genuine smile but certainly didn't want anyone blowing false hope my way.

I was in luck. Lindsey wasn't pretending to be nice because my circumstances were bleak, she was just plain nice. There was no false bravado, and her smile was infectious. Her fun sense of humor was an added bonus, shattering the tension that had been building in my system since entering the hospital and being asked about my living will.

I could only imagine how difficult and somber Lindsey's job must be, dealing with people fighting cancer all day long and relaying bad news to their family members. I was glad to share in her sense of humor and easy-going personality, which relaxed me immediately. I had been expecting someone with the sobriety of an Old West undertaker, but Lindsey was a much-needed ray of sunshine in my world.

She quickly reviewed my medical records and said, "Tell me your story. Do you smoke or drink excessively? Tell me how you found out about this tumor."

I began to relay my very boring story of how I had gone to my primary care doctor with bronchitis, was referred to a podiatrist to remove a ganglion cyst, and ended up with cancer. No great punch line. No dramatic history. I was the picture of health for thirty-seven years and ended up with a rare sarcoma after my first visit to the outpatient clinic.

The extensive black, blue, and purple bruising on my leg had penetrated to my kneecap and was now radiating red streaks in every direction. I was probably the only one in the room who didn't realize how serious the staph infection was at the original site of excision. I knew my foot hurt enough to validate my Vicodin prescription, but I didn't know exactly why. After all, this was my first surgical experience. I thought everything was normal.

As Lindsey continued to look at my leg, she said something I will never forget if I live to be two hundred years old. "After you finish your initial treatment here, we will be examining you once every quarter for many, many years to come."

For several moments time stood still, while hot tears began to flood my eyes, pouring down my cheeks as relief washed over my entire being. Lindsey was the first sarcoma specialist to give me a good, solid dose of hope. She was talking to me as if I would be around for years to come.

God had answered my prayers. A huge burden was immediately lifted from my shoulders, and I was speechless. The breath that I didn't even know I was holding was suddenly released as tears continued flowing down my face.

Diana began to explain to Lindsey that she was the first medically trained person with any level of sarcoma expertise to give us hope. Many others were giving us bad news, telling us this was a rare cancer that was difficult to fight, but Lindsey had given us hope. In that instant I was dancing on air.

Lindsey looked at me with great compassion. "We see this stuff all the time. It's no big deal."

I was part of the crowd, the sarcoma crowd with the specialist who knew just what to do. I was elated.

The door opened, and a physician's assistant came in to look at my leg. He immediately noticed the staph infection then asked about the crooked pattern of the incision. We joked about it, because there was nothing either one of us could do about the jagged, infected scar on my leg. Obviously, this was the least of my concerns.

The physician's assistant looked at me and said, "Tell me your story. Do you smoke or drink excessively?" I told him I didn't do either and began relaying my lackluster ganglion cyst story all over again. He made some more notes on my chart, and we waited together for the doctor's arrival.

The room was getting crowded, my makeup had already been destroyed, and my leg was throbbing, but I was full to the rim with absolute joy and great expectation.

At M.D. Anderson, when you request to be seen, they review all of your results surrounding your diagnosis. Once these results are verified by a second and third consenting opinion, you are assigned to a specialized team of doctors who map out a strategy for your specific needs. Since M.D. Anderson is a teaching hospital in the University of Texas system, there are always new faces assisting the doctors (interns, physicians assistants, fellows), but your assigned team of doctors stays the same unless a new symptom is revealed or one of the doctors leaves the hospital.

Dr. Yasko was the original oncologist who had been assigned to my team. As he opened the exam room door, my hopes and expectations shot through the roof, and I could almost hear the "Hallelujah Chorus" playing in the background. I was finally going to get some long-awaited answers from an actual, bona fide sarcoma oncologist.

Dr. Yasko smiled warmly and extended his hand to me. I smiled back while shaking his hand, knowing that today was going to be my first step toward recovery.

"Tell me your story," he said. "Do you smoke or drink excessively?"

I couldn't stop laughing. I told him I was going to record my story on a small tape so I could re-play it every time someone asked me how I discovered my cancer. My diagnosis was not going to be the next Sunday night movie on prime time television. I was growing tired of repeating it. I wanted to know what I needed to do to get rid of the cancer. Still, I repeated my story for the third time in as many hours, hoping the third time would be the charm and the doctor would help me devise a quick plan for treatment. I still had yet to learn that *quick* and *cancer* never go together.

In one of the greatest art masterpieces I have ever seen, Dr. Yasko began to sketch the details of my case on the crisp white paper lining covering the exam table.

"There are three things that we look for when evaluating cancer. First we look for depth. The depth of your tumor was not deep by our standards. The fact that you could see it with your naked eye tells us that it was superficial by our standards. It is rare to have this type of cancer in the extremities and even more rare to be able to see it so clearly with the naked eye."

"The second thing we look for is size. The size of your

tumor is three centimeters. If it was five centimeters or more, we would have to start chemotherapy immediately."

I looked at Dr. Yasko and said, "Yay me!"

"Yes, that's great," he said. "And you even get to keep your hair." We both laughed.

"The third thing we look for is the grade. On a scale of one to four, yours is a four, meaning it is the most aggressive, most likely to recur, and most likely to move to another part of the body. But you have two of the three things going for you."

I laughed as I told him that rare and aggressive were both character traits I understood very well.

I was so relieved to know what I was up against. I was grinning from ear to ear like a Cheshire cat, knowing that even in the worst of circumstances, God had carried me through my cancer initiation. He didn't send angels to escort me; he showed up himself.

As the news of my extremely rare and aggressive cancer was relayed to me, I began to not only understand but live the true meaning of grace. There was every reason for me to die. But God.

Psalm 118:17–18 says, "I shall not die, but live, and declare the works of the Lord. The Lord has chastened me severely, But He has not given me over to death."

Leiomyosarcoma was not known for responding to treatment, but the Healer was passing by. I was reaching for the hem of his garment, and I knew he would not leave me behind (Matthew 9:20–22).

My mind was reeling with this new heady excitement launched by these brilliant doctors telling me that I was going to *live*. It took me more than a few moments to shove my own thoughts to the side and realize that the doctor was still patiently explaining my sarcoma to me in vivid detail.

By the time I came down from the clouds, Dr. Yasko was explaining things that patients normally wonder but are too afraid to ask. They were not planning to cut my leg off. I might have another surgery to remove any remaining cancer cells and re-construct my leg, which would be a massive undertaking. But I would keep my leg. My prognosis was very good, which was music to my ears. If my leg hadn't felt like it was in a vice, I'm pretty sure I would have danced for joy right there in front of God and everyone.

Radiation treatments were at the top of the laundry list of recommendations suggested by my team of doctors. Since my original surgery was not conducted by an oncologist, and the MRI showed no clear margins, a second, more extensive surgery might be necessary after radiation to eliminate any remaining cancer cells.

"Clear margins" is a term oncologists use when they are looking at slides of cancer cells. When you cut out a cancerous tumor, you need to cut a surrounding border of healthy cells to ensure all of the cancer was removed. If there are cancer cells from one end of the slide to the other, then you don't have clear margins, and it is likely some cancer remains behind in the body.

The physician's assistant began removing my sutures from the site of the excision. He couldn't find all of the sutures, so he used a scalpel to dig them out of the jagged pattern cut during the original surgery. By this time my leg was on fire, and I was ready to go back to the hotel and pack my leg with ice. I'd had all the fun I needed for one day.

But before heading back, we had lunch plans with some very dear friends, the Leibmans. I went inside the restaurant alone, hobbling on my crutches as my foot continued to throb. I felt as if I was dragging a boat anchor, yet my heart was as light as a feather. Diana was still talking on the phone in the car, trying to find an apartment to rent for the coming weeks of radiation.

A few minutes later Diana appeared at our table with Dodie Osteen, the mother of Joel Osteen, the senior pastor of Lakewood Church in Houston. Dodie attended school with my dad, so my family has known the Osteens for many years. Dodie is a cancer survivor, so it was especially nice when she came over to our table and graciously offered to pray for me.

"I know you are probably wondering *why me*. Why did this happen to me?"

I looked at her and said, "Dodie, why *not* me?"

I think she was surprised at my answer, but she smiled as Diana said, "She has that Hagee fight in her. With God's help we are going to beat this thing." Dodie nodded in agreement and prayed over my leg for complete healing. It was a delicious lunch.

That week I endured many tests that pushed my body to new limits. There were CT scans, blood tests, x-rays, MRIs, you name it. I had turned into a human lab rat. I was finishing one of my last tests when the technician looked at my chart and did a double take. "Is John Hagee your brother?" I laughed (to keep from crying) and told her that he was my dad. I was hoping she listened to him on the radio and didn't watch him on TV, or else I looked worse than I thought.

If you have never experienced the adventure of extensive medical testing, let me explain what it is like. The CT scan, computed tomography (or "CAT scan" as it is often called), is a painless medical test that helps doctors see the inside of your body with more clarity than an x-ray. According to www.radiologyinfo.org, "CT imaging uses special x-ray equipment to produce multiple images or pictures of the inside of the body and a computer to join them together in cross-sectional views of the area being studied. The images can them be examined on a computer monitor or printed."

In layman's terms, you show up at the counter where the nurse presents you with a not-so-delicious bottle of chilled, liquid chalk that has some type of vanilla or berry flavor attached to it and expects you to drink the entire thing in thirty minutes without tossing your cookies on the floor. After two hours and four bottles of satisfying and very filling liquid chalk, you are ready for your CT scan. The scan is painless. You are put on a table that takes multiple pictures of the area in high definition; you joke with the technicians about wanting a six-pack of nutritious liquid chalk to take home and enjoy over the weekend; and you are ready to go. The radiologist will read the pictures and tell your oncologist if anything noteworthy appears.

The table they lay you on for the CT is small, and the thin circular camera quickly glides over your body. Claustrophobics have no problem here. The MRI (Magnetic Resonance Imaging) is a whole different ballgame. Thankfully, here you only have to inject the dye instead of drinking liquid berry-flavored chalk that settles into your stomach like a vat of glue.

According to www.radiologyinfo.com, "MR imaging uses

a powerful magnetic field, radio waves and a computer to produce detailed pictures of organs, soft tissues, bone and virtually all other internal body structures. The images can then be examined on a computer monitor or printed. MRI does not use ionizing radiation (x-rays). Detailed MR images allow physicians to better evaluate parts of the body and certain diseases that may not be assessed adequately with other imaging methods such as x-ray, ultrasound or … CAT scanning."

If you have ever thought about being claustrophobic, this will bring out the very best in you.

The MRI machine is a narrow bed that shoots into something the size of a large Tylenol capsule. It is sort of like putting a human body into a pixie stick or sticking an adult giraffe inside a Pacer with no sun roof. As the table beneath you starts sliding into the black hole, you are hoping you can get both butt cheeks inside without scraping your nose on the top of the tube. I am only five feet two inches tall and not a very large person, yet I am still a snug fit for the inside of this oversized camera, which takes high definition pictures of my ankle and lower body in order to see how widespread the cancer is.

My favorite part is when the radiology technician says, "Please don't move for the next hour and a half."

Where am I going to go if I am stuffed like a human sausage into this enormous machine? Even if I wanted to move, the most I could do is blink or perhaps slightly twitch my leg.

As the technician leaves the room, you begin to slide into the belly of the camera for a long winter's nap, only to be interrupted by something that sounds like a combination of machine gun artillery and jack hammers playing in tandem. Sadly enough, since I live with two young, active girls and a multitude of pets, I can sleep through this symphonic melody until the technicians come in and wake me up to inject the dye.

During this long week of testing, we were privileged to meet the much-acclaimed Dr. Benjamin, head of the sarcoma department and top recommendation of Capitol Hill. Everyone who knew him revered him to the fullest extent and referred to him with great respect as "the man." We were not on his agenda, and for him to even consider consulting with us was a miracle all its own.

In fact, his nurse very kindly told us that since we were not already on his schedule, we probably would not be able to visit with him at all. The oncologists at M.D. Anderson have rigorous schedules that are completely maxed out until late in the evening, so it would be a huge honor just to consult with him. God was good, and we were granted great favor once again (Psalm 30:5).

At 7:00 p.m. one evening, after his normal clinic hours, Dr. Benjamin took the time to review my chart. He came in and greeted me like I was the most important person he had seen all day.

Dr. Benjamin was brilliant, kind, and exceptionally humble. Buttons from his patients covered his white lab coat in an array of rainbow colors and varied sentiments. One that stood out for me said in bright red letters, "sarcoma sucks." I laughed when I read that, and he said it was one of his favorite buttons too.

I was stunned to find that he had already reviewed the test results performed throughout the week, including some that had just been completed only moments before. He was already aware of the details of my case, even though I wasn't his patient, and very graciously started answering our seemingly endless litany of questions.

When we came up for air, he gave me the news I had been waiting all week to hear; the cancer had not spread throughout my body. Thank you, God. I had just walked to his office from the final set of tests and was already listening to the results. My mind went into overdrive at this wonderfully liberating discovery. Once again, everything in the universe ceased to exist as I absorbed this overwhelming bit of exceptional news.

I was amazed at the efficiency of this life-saving medical metropolis, and my heart danced knowing that, once again, I was in the right place at the right time. God had remained faithful to the promises he had given me, and the good news just kept pouring in (Psalm 107:1–9). Before I was even born, he knew I would one day face this monumental problem, and he had begun to prepare me for it before I even knew what leiomyosarcoma was (Psalm 139:15–16).

Diana told Dr. Benjamin that her sister had passed away at eighteen with neomyosarcoma, so she wanted to understand what our next steps would be. You could see a bewildered look come over Dr. Benjamin's face. He explained that this type of cancer is so rare it should never occur twice in the same family.

Anyone sharing my bloodline could not possibly have the same type of sarcoma. Diana quickly explained that she was my step-mother, and, noting that we would not be the first ones in history to mess up this theory, Dr. Benjamin quickly went on to describe my possible treatment scenarios.

I would probably need five weeks of radiation, which would mean coming for treatment five days a week in Houston for five solid weeks.

The helium balloon that had my emotions flying high immediately exploded. What about my job? What about my kids? What about my dogs and my house? Who would take care of everything if I was away that long? How could we survive on only one income for that length of time? How long would it take me to get back on my feet at work?

Since I am a loan officer and originate home loans, I work on commission. This meant if I was not working, I was not making money. What was I going to do? A whole new set of questions flooded my brain, and I could once again feel the raindrops starting to pound my parade.

Diana could see the concern flashing in my eyes and began to relay them to Dr. Benjamin. He leaned over my wheelchair and looked me right in the eyes. In one of the most gracious and loving statements I have ever heard, he said, "Tish, you are worth it. Whatever it takes, you are worth it."

I stood up from my wheelchair as best I could, and he hugged me with great compassion. Whatever it took, I had to make this work. I was just beginning to understand that the only thing I was going to be able to focus on in the immediate future was my health. There was no quick fix here.

Every day would be a fight for survival. My dad always says, "You either get the cancer, or the cancer gets you." I didn't want the cancer to win (Exodus 14:14).

It was the end of June, and the end of a long week of physically and mentally exhausting tests. I was grateful to be with a team of exceptional experts that were assimilated to attack my disease without intimidation or apology.

After this fact-finding mission, I had a much greater understanding of what I was up against and was now ready to fight more than ever. Hillary Clinton might only need a village, but I needed an entire army. I needed God's army (Matthew 9:20–22).

> Oh, taste and see that the Lord is good; blessed is the man who trusts in Him! Oh, fear the Lord, you his saints! There is no want to those who fear him. The young lions lack and suffer hunger; but those who seek the Lord shall not lack any good thing.
>
> Psalm 34:8–10

My first night in Houston, I had seen the fear of death rear its ugly head in my hotel room. Now it was time to practice a healthy fear of God, for I wanted to lack nothing. I wanted to use this time for my own personal rejuvenation so that at the end of this cancer journey, I would not only be a stronger person physically and spiritually, but I could reach out to those around me going through similar trials and offer the same encouragement I had received from survivors around the globe immediately following my diagnosis when my world seemed to be crumbling before my very eyes. Now that every inch of my body had been tested, poked, and x-rayed, it was time to head home and wrap my arms around my babies, which were my true reason for living.

Good Staff, Bad Staph, Ugly Staph

When I returned home, it was as if flyers had rained out of airplanes all over the United States announcing that I had been diagnosed with cancer. I had previously done my best to keep a tight rein on the news, not knowing the parameters of what I was facing.

Of course, I knew before I left for Houston that I had failed miserably at keeping this news quarantined. I assumed that most people who knew me on a first-name basis knew about my diagnosis by the time I left. However, by the time I came back from Houston, I had become the topic of conversation *du jour* among groups of people that were totally foreign to me. Suddenly I was deluged by emails, calls, letters, and messages pouring in from people I went to kindergarten with, people I hadn't spoken to in years, people from far and near, and people I had never met.

There were gift baskets and packages, books, t-shirts, pamphlets, vitamins, bottled water, herbs, and health magazines especially designed for cancer patients. It was as if the Hoover Dam had exploded and thousands of people were sending me their love and support from all over the world.

My army had arrived in all shapes and sizes and from all corners of the universe. It was completely unexpected and overwhelming in a way that I had not experienced before. I felt like I was being crushed with good news and support at every turn. Could this many people truly care about me? Strangers and friends alike were coming out of the wood-work to help me, to pray for me, to encourage me, to fast for me, to bring my family meals, to help me at work, to do anything it took to reach out and help me.

This was the grandest and most incredible display I had ever witnessed. It was beyond my wildest imagination and far exceeded anything I could have hoped for. People were stop-ping their own lives to reach out to meet my every need. We overuse the word awesome on a daily basis, but this truly was awesome in every sense of the word. It touched my heart, as if I were dying of thirst and thousands of people began to show up at my door with their last glass of water just for me.

I had to keep pinching myself to believe it was really hap-pening to *me*. I was like the woman in 1 Kings 17:11–16 who filled up every pot in her house with oil. There were no more pots to fill. It was incredibly moving and humbling at the same time.

Here I had kept the news to myself so I could fully grasp the meaning of how cancer would be affecting my body, and thousands of people were just waiting to show me unrelent-ing and unconditional love and support. It was an amazing demonstration of friendship on the highest level. Acts of genuine caring were saturating every moment of my day and consuming my thoughts, which was a welcome change from the chaos that had reigned there just a few days before.

Again, I had to ask why? Why did I deserve this outpouring of love (3 John 2)? I am happy to go visit sick friends or family members in the hospital or take meals to people who are recovering, but I am not comfortable with other people coming by my house to do the same for me.

The news continued rushing through the country like a wild brushfire, and more people were beginning to contact me every day. By this time I could no longer keep up with my email, so I started a blog called "Tish's Triumphs." Every few days I would update the site with news from my doctors, how my treatment was going, or some great lesson I picked up in the process.

I wanted the entries to help someone else in need or lift someone's spirits that might be going through a similar challenge. I really needed to help other people and didn't want to wait until I was feeling better to start. Besides, no one could tell me with any certainty when I would ever be well again, or if this cancer would plague me for the rest of my life. The time for action was now. I was too tired to physically go out and help people, so I filled my blog.

The blog address was spread quickly, and complete strangers were responding on a daily basis. One lady said she had been suicidal because things weren't going well for her. After reading my blog she realized that her life wasn't really that bad and was certainly worth saving. She had started reading the Bible again and praying. She no longer had suicidal tendencies.

Another mother said it gave her hope for her son's upcoming treatment. Still another man said he had started reading the Bible again with his family and was fully expecting God to heal him of this terrible disease we shared. God was sending people my way from every walk of life. These people needed help overcoming tremendous trials in their own lives, not necessarily healing. It was wonderful to share the Source of all hope and to take the focus off my own situation for just a brief moment.

I knew this was just one of the reasons God trusted me with this most rare disease. I began craving opportunities to reach out and touch the lives of others who were without hope or joy, who needed new direction, or just wanted a friendly ear to bend. I knew now that if I had a common cancer that wasn't quite so deadly or aggressive, people might be less likely to listen and more apt to credit the doctors with my fantastic results.

But I had a sarcoma that affected four out of every one million sarcoma patients and did not respond to treatment. I had better odds of winning the mega lottery or getting struck by lightning. If I was completely healed of an incurable disease like this, surely all of the honor would go to the Great Physician himself (Zechariah 4:6).

If I didn't have cancer, I could never sympathize with the people who were now contacting me faster than I could respond. I would not know how to relate to them or comfort them in their greatest hour of need. Now I was a part of the cancer club, and I completely understood. I was a card-carrying member of a society to which no one wants to pay dues.

Having the opportunity to reach out and encourage others was extraordinary. It made me feel in an odd way like my cancer was a gift. It was a resource that gave me secret passage into the lives of others, a way to encourage a group

I had unexpectedly joined. It was spectacular to be able to share true stories of God's mercy in my own life with those who needed to hear it most.

During the July 4th weekend, the pain in my leg became unbearable. Dr. Kalter, the oncologist in San Antonio who was monitoring my wound, directed me to the local emergency room. The ER was packed. Since I was not pouring blood from my head and didn't have a gunshot wound, I knew I would not be a priority.

My leg was throbbing with every beat of my heart and the hospital administrator didn't want me to prop it up. She looked at me with disdain and growled, "I don't want to spread anything contagious from your leg." Without missing a beat I replied with a fake but sweet smile on my face, "I don't believe cancer is contagious, so you're in luck." I kept my oversized foot propped up, daring her to touch it. My "nice" had been used up.

Johnny Gross, the minister of music at our church, met us at the door. It was great to see a familiar face. Since all of my previous treatments had been in Houston, it was unusual to see anyone I recognized at the hospital. So we did what everyone does in the emergency room; we waited, and then we waited some more. Throb. Throb. Throb.

When my name was finally called, the ER doctor determined I had a severe staph infection. It had been weeks since my surgery, and I wondered why I had seen so many doctors who recognized that my purple and grossly-swollen leg was infected with staph, and yet this was the first one to clue me in. Then it hit me—cancer trumps staph. I had been treating the greater of two evils.

It was quickly determined that my leg needed to be treated with vancomycin, the strongest antibiotic available in an IV. It is so strong that once it is used in an IV, the tubes have to be thrown away because it burns holes in the tubing. Knowing this wasn't exactly comforting, but if the vancomycin would reduce the infection without burning my leg off, I was willing to give it a try. So I waited a little more until they set up my IV and prepared my leg to feel a great surge of relief as the antibiotics filtered through my body.

Unfortunately, my body was not in love with this particular brand of medicine and reacted horribly. Within minutes my entire body started itching uncontrollably and a rash broke out all over my back and arms. The doctor decided to stop this antibiotic and shoot some Benadryl through my IV tube to stop the itching.

The two medicines collided in my body like a giant train wreck, and I felt like my lungs were collapsing. I couldn't breathe. I thought I was dying. My eyes were huge and watering as I started gasping for air, wanting desperately to hurt the person who had just pumped me full of meds that were obviously deflating my lungs.

There was only enough oxygen to gasp out, "I can't breathe. I can't breathe." At that exact moment, Diana was standing by the side of my bed talking to my dad on the cell phone. All he could hear on his side of the conversation was, "I can't breathe." Talk about bad timing.

The doctor kept assuring me that my oxygenation level was at 95 percent, but his calm demeanor was doing nothing to placate me. I wanted to choke him with his tie and see how he liked not being able to breathe. I kept motioning with frenzied hands that I couldn't breathe, but every part of me wanted to scream, "I'm not going to survive cancer to be killed by antibiotics in the emergency room! Somebody help me out over here! Get me some air, pronto!"

After what seemed like an eternity (about a minute or so), the medicines settled in my system, and I could finally breathe again. My body was tied in knots. Every part of my abdomen was cramping, and I felt as if I had been stabbed a thousand times. My breathing was labored, and I was lying on my hospital bed like a limp rag doll, feeling like an eighteen-wheeler had just run over me then backed up his truck and come back for round two. Right about this time, my dad showed up.

I couldn't move. It hurt to even open my eyeballs. I wanted someone to give me a morphine pump and wake me up in three or four days when the pain had subsided and my leg was no longer infected. That didn't happen.

A few hours later, I was admitted to the hospital for four days of IV antibiotics. Happy Fourth of July!

The nurses were phenomenal at the Methodist Hospital in San Antonio. The food was great. The room was huge. My friends and family could come and see me. After I got over the reaction to the meds and was introduced to a new antibiotic, life was good.

My vitals did not have to be checked during this hospital stay, so I could sleep like a baby, completely uninterrupted all night long. All I had to do was sleep and wake up completely refreshed. Ahhhhh! But all good things must come to an end, and four days later I was released with an almost normal-sized foot barely showing signs of discoloration.

The following week I confirmed with Dr. Kalter that the staph infection I was admitted to the hospital with was a blessing in disguise. The white blood cells in my leg were fighting both the infection and the cancer cells. God was good. He was fighting my disease in ways I didn't even know were possible.

On July 12, 2006, I emailed pictures of my ankle to Lindsey, the sarcoma nurse at M.D. Anderson whom I had met during my initial visit. Even after my Fourth of July hospital stint, the doctors at M.D. Anderson were concerned about the amount of infection remaining in my foot. They wanted to see my leg again to surmise if a second surgery was warranted to remove any remaining cancer cells. It was highly likely that the cancer had spread throughout my body via the blood that traveled up my infected leg after the original excision. So, off to Houston I went for another round of tests and exams.

I thought my leg was looking better by the minute, but evidently what the doctors saw upon my arrival concerned them. The dead ("necrotic") tissue surrounding the original surgical wound was becoming more apparent. If a second surgery was needed, the oncologists said it would be a "big deal," combining two surgeries into one. I was familiar with the buy one, get one free service at the mall, but I was pretty sure I didn't want to get the same type of deal from my oncological surgeon.

If this second surgery came to fruition, it would be a massive undertaking that would take several teams of doctors to reconstruct my leg. The oncologist would perform the first surgery, removing all areas potentially infected by any remaining cancer. The second surgery would be conducted by a plastic surgeon, who would reconstruct my lower leg using muscle and tissue from my upper leg.

I had never had plastic surgery at that point in my life and was relatively certain I wanted my first plastic surgery experience to be for cosmetic reasons and not to reconstruct my leg after removing a cancerous tumor. I wanted something to be thinner, perkier, or much more beautiful, not just functional. But under the current circumstances, I was willing to make an exception. Whatever it was going to take, I was ready.

The doctors at M.D. Anderson made some notes on my chart and sent me home to heal for a while before returning for more observation and testing. They are very good at the wait-and-see approach, so I was sent home to do my least favorite thing—wait.

I was told to soak my leg and scrub off all dead tissue surrounding the original site of excision. Not an ideal way for a gal to spend an evening, but it meant keeping my leg, so I kept scrubbing with a smile on my face, thinking of how wonderful my leg would be when it was no longer reptilian looking.

One of my favorite decadent pleasures is to have a spa pedicure, which involves scraping the dead skin off your feet. Since I constantly run around my house without shoes on, I always have plenty of dead skin. I was ready to soak my leg and scrape this skin off my ankle just like I did at home when I couldn't make it to the spa for my feet. Boy, what an idiot. Why did I ever think that the million and one nerve endings on the top of my foot that had been heightened by recent surgery would be as painless as a pedicure?

A few Sundays later, David Ring was the guest speaker at our church. David is a motivational Christian speaker from Jonesboro, Arkansas, who has valiantly fought cerebral palsy his entire life. He was orphaned at fourteen when his mother died and has overcome obstacles that would completely debilitate a lesser man. David travels all over the country sharing his story, encouraging others, and recounting the blessings in his own life.

I had been out of touch for a while, so it was a pleasant surprise to see David when I walked into my dad's office in the back of the church building. David has an innate ability to put a smile on anyone's face, and today would be no exception. It was great to see him!

After the service I would be heading back to M.D. Anderson for more testing the following day, and my body was growing weary from all the poking, prodding, and constant traveling.

I was ready for a break. I just wanted to climb in a cave and take a nap for a week or two and then start over on the tests, X-rays, and MRIs that my doctors seemed so fond of repeating every time I saw them.

Just as I was beginning to mentally prepare myself for the tests that were coming the following day, and sink into physical and emotional exhaustion, I saw David looking at me with a smile that radiated from his heart. My ailments just started a few weeks ago, and here I was thinking about my own exhaustion (2 Corinthians 12: 9–10). Shame on me!

David came up and wrapped his arms around me. "Tish,

your dad has told me what you are going through, and I want you to know that I'm praying for you."

I looked into his sweet face and said with total confidence, "David, everything is going to be all right."

"I know it is," he said. "I know it is."

David had suffered greatly every day of his life, and here *he* was praying for *me*. It was difficult for David to speak, write, or move quickly. He stamps the signature line on his checks because it takes too long to write his name.

All of these difficulties with his own daily endeavors, and he was taking no thought for himself. David Ring was thinking only of praying for *my* healing. I was humbled to the core. God had sent another messenger to remind me that he was the fourth man in my fire (Daniel 3:25).

David's message was entitled, "Living Above the Storm." I have heard him speak many times, but that particular Sunday the sermon was perfect for me. The point was how God's grace can help you through the toughest storm of your life. If you aren't currently in a storm, you are headed for one or you just got out of one. No one escapes the storms of life, and everyone has a story.

That evening I made the three-hour trek to Houston with Diana one more time. I took no thought for my physical exhaustion (Proverbs 17:22). If David Ring could smile his way through life, so could I.

As I wheeled myself toward the sarcoma wing the following morning, my leg was still in a great deal of pain. Regardless, I felt blessed beyond measure (Job 10:12). If you ever feel like you are having a bad day or you are the only one suffering in the world, take a drive to your local cancer ward. Take a peek inside. It is a tiny glimpse inside hell.

A cancer ward is chock-full of people who give suffering a new meaning. Real-life cancer doesn't look anywhere near as glamorous as the movies. Inside a cancer hospital you will no longer feel badly about your current circumstances. Your perspective on life and health, gratitude and death will be much different. You will no longer dread that milestone birthday, but you will embrace each day for the true gift that it is. Cancer gives you a new respect for what is truly important in life.

These flashes of gratitude began to race through my mind as I found myself once again waiting for my name to be called and my appointment with the oncologist to begin.

I was now a sarcoma veteran, and happy for the opportunity to chat with new patients. I always do my best to offer a friendly smile laced with hope. I tell them how I rejoice by choice every morning when I open my eyes (Psalm 100). After relaying my own personal story, I tell them about the favor God has rained down on my life, favor that is free to anyone for the asking.

There is an instant bond among cancer patients. You know that you may never see each other again, but you have walked a mile in each other's shoes. You understand something in the very depths of your soul that others cannot truly grasp. The cancer patients in the waiting room may not have one other person in their life who understands where they have been or where they are going, but you have a silent and heart-rending knowledge of the path they are on because it is disturbingly similar to your own.

Smile a While

Laughter truly is the best medicine (Isaiah 55:12). Every time I walked (or rolled my wheelchair) into the exam room, I made it a point to smile at everyone and laugh at myself and my circumstances as much as possible. I wanted to find the good in my situation and rise above the grim circumstances that I knew to be the truth.

I was not denying that I had a problem. I just wanted to see any light in my temporarily dark tunnel. When you aim for the light, the dark shadows around you begin to disappear. Besides, cancer is very expensive, and smiling doesn't even involve a co-pay.

Franklin D. Roosevelt said, "There is nothing to fear except fear itself." That is so true. The fear can kill you faster than the cancer. I had no reason to fear (Philippians 4:4–7) and much to live for.

Cancer is a stressful, emotional game as much as a physical challenge. If you don't have a positive attitude and focus on the good things in your life, the cancer will destroy you from the inside out. There are days that drain every drop of energy just to get out of bed for five minutes. But you have to be grateful for those five minutes. You are still alive, and with cancer, it is a race against the clock. Every minute is precious. Time is an invaluable commodity that money cannot buy and no friend can give you (Psalm 31:14–16).

I laughed every chance I got, with every doctor and patient who would listen. I was not disrespectful or nonchalant. I respected the toll cancer has taken on so many millions of lives and the severity to which it could ravage a body in such a short period of time, how it could destroy lives and homes. However, I knew it was imminently important for my survival to bring humor to the very sober place at which I had arrived in my life (Psalm 5:11–12).

My doctors were exceptional, extraordinary on every level, yet they remained humble in the face of severe adversity as they treated me in a series of completely selfless acts. There was no great award ceremony for them at the end if I lived, or if I was happy with my treatment. They didn't receive a bonus on their paycheck if my radiation worked. Yet they continued coming to work each day for the greater good of their patients. I could not have been more grateful or more humbled by their unrelenting pursuit of a cure for my disease.

My doctors were constantly smiling and greeting me warmly, as if they were old friends who genuinely cared about my well being. Why shouldn't I return that smile and share some hope with them too? After all, they *chose* to be there.

There are no paltry words of gratitude great enough or sincere enough to even begin to thank someone for not only saving but extending your life.

These doctors provided me with cutting edge treatment,

endless hours of consultation both in person and on the phone, and a billion tests for every inch of my body. All I had to offer was my smile. This was no quid pro quo. They were definitely getting the short end of the stick.

There were many days that laughter helped me get through that twenty-three-hour period between treatments, and the seemingly endless hours of waiting. I spent so many hours in the waiting room that I probably could have perfected a third hobby or learned a tenth language, had my own seat monogrammed or tried out thirty new hair dos. As I began to become more accustomed to the quality time I was spending in the waiting rooms, I began to pray that God would direct the people to me who needed to hear words of hope (John 10:9–10).

My oncologist, Dr. Yasko, began my next visit by poking my ankle. "Does this hurt?"

I laughed, as if it would make a difference. Wow! We were going to try something new today—poking the ol' ankle.

My leg had been treated by so many doctors from San Antonio to Houston that at this point all I could do was joke about how sexy it looked. My leg had disgusting dead and peeling skin, nasty razor stubble that I could do nothing about under the circumstances, and dry legs that would rival any alligator. I was a real looker, ready for the runway.

Dr. Yasko thought my foot looked great, much improved since our last visit. I was not going to make it into the next Sports Illustrated Swimsuit Edition, but the infection and swelling were gone along with the black and blue bruising. There was only one piece of dead tissue in the center of the wound site, and the doctors were sure this would dry up and peel away. No one believed a second surgery would be necessary. There was much to smile about (Psalm 28:6–9).

My appointment with the oncologist was over, and Diana once again pushed my wheelchair through the hospital corridors and out to the car. I was elated that my leg was healing so completely but was almost ashamed at my own personal celebration as I noticed the numerous patients surrounding me who were missing limbs, shrouded in a dark cloud of pain. It was a sight I would never get used to. Each time I saw these patients, I was grateful all over again for my body parts.

Thank you, God, that no matter how much my leg hurts, I get to keep my leg! The throbbing of my leg was a constant reminder that it was still attached to my body. Before my diagnosis I had wished my legs were thinner and could fit into cute shorts and fun summer dresses. Now I was just glad to have two legs, no matter what size they were. What a difference a day makes.

On my way out to the parking lot, I continued my visual perusal of the patients who, once again, filled every possible corridor and passageway. I was ready to take a break from this place that seemed to completely drain me both physically and emotionally, if only for the day. I wanted to recline my seat in the air-conditioned confines of the car with people who were completely healthy and talked about the weather. Looking around at those suffering from various types of cancer was a constant reminder of where I might be headed. It was a harsh and constant reality, and I was ready for just a touch of fantasy.

We were finally back in the safety of our car, and it was time to head for home and share the good news. The bad news I was hit with during my initial diagnosis was hard to hand out, but good news is like cash money. Everybody wants to share it.

I was amazed at the masses of people who turned out to help me after my diagnosis, but that was just the tip of the iceberg. I was not on the Titanic after all. The outpouring of God's blessings in my life had only just begun, and there was no end in sight. I was constantly reminded of every good and perfect gift. As I continued to thank him, he continued to show up in person to fight my battles (Psalm 121).

Keeping the "RAD" in Radiation

My medical team at M.D. Anderson had already spent several days mapping out my treatment schedule during my initial week of testing. I spent time in the hospital undergoing a strict regimen of antibiotics in the hope of ridding my body of the far-reaching staph infection and was now ready for the radiation treatments I had discussed with Dr. Benjamin. It was time for me to move from the care of my oncologist to my radiologist. Dr. Ballo was the radiologist assigned to my case, so I began to mentally prepare for radiation, though I truly had no idea what the process would entail or how my body would respond.

What exactly was radiation? How would I feel? How would I look? Would my hair fall out? Would I be nauseous all the time? Would I start to look like Sigorney Weaver in the movie *Alien*? How long would the treatment last, and would it work? Didn't the doctors say that leiomyosarcoma doesn't respond to treatment?

Even though my sarcoma was not one slated to respond to treatment, the medical team decided to give it a try.

Five weeks seemed like an eternity to be away from my home, my job, and my family. Five weeks in the grand scheme of life is not a long time, but I didn't want to be away from my girls or from work for that long. When you are talking about cancer, you never know how much time you have or how long the course of your treatment will take. You don't know if your treatment will work tomorrow or ten years from now. You don't know much of anything, so you take one day at a time. Matthew 6:33–34 says:

> But seek ye first the kingdom of God and His righteousness, and all these things shall be added to you. Therefore do not worry about tomorrow, for tomorrow will worry about its own things. Sufficient for the day is its own trouble.

No matter how unpleasant, I was ready for whatever my radiologist recommended. Dr. Ballo had witnessed firsthand the rampant staph infection in my leg during one of my initial visits to M.D. Anderson and now, just a few short weeks later, was elated to see that it had healed enough to begin daily radiation treatments.

I loved my appointments with Dr. Ballo. There are some people in this life who have the uncanny ability to make you feel right at home the moment you meet them. I greatly appreciated his warm, friendly smile and wonderful, dry sense of humor. Of course, you can't really be Chuckles the

Clown working at a cancer hospital, but we tried to introduce humor to each visit.

As with my other doctors, I wanted to laugh as much as possible, and Dr. Ballo was a kind and gracious participant in my humor-based treatment regimen. He reiterated that I would need five weeks of radiation, starting July 31, 2006. He would meet with me once a week to track my progress and answer any questions. If I missed any of my appointments, the hospital policy dictated he could choose to discontinue my treatments.

M.D. Anderson has people waiting to get in the door from all corners of the globe, so I wanted to make sure the doctors knew the extent of my gratitude for their time and attention. I would be there each morning with bells on. These guys were literally saving my life. That was no joke, but certainly something worth smiling about.

Since my original excision had not completely sealed, Dr. Ballo warned me that the wound on my right ankle would probably re-open at some point during the radiation and start oozing from the inside. As attractive as that sounded, I was ready to begin treatment and get on with the show. Let the games begin.

By mid-July I was getting tattooed "markings" at the hospital, which are permanent black dots that precisely guide the technicians as they line up the radiation machines. The radiologist tells the physician's assistant exactly where to tattoo the dots so that each treatment is precisely executed. There is no room for error. You cannot radiate only 99 percent of the cancer (Psalm 30:5).

I asked for a more decorative tattoo option, something colorful and floral instead of an assortment of black dots, but that was the extent of the tattoo artistry at M.D. Anderson. We were on a healing mission, and the dots would do the trick. I jokingly told the assistant I would be back for an upgrade after my treatments were over.

It was important for me to let every single person involved in my cancer journey know that the joy of the Lord was my strength and that I would eventually defeat my cancer. I was not afraid. I was grateful for every single day, and in short order I would be more than a conqueror (Psalm 30:10–12).

The radiation treatments were measured in millimeters. X-rays would be taken once a week to illustrate my progress. If the x-ray was done incorrectly, the radiologist would order new ones, even if it was off by a fraction of a millimeter. I was grateful for the exactness and certainty of this science because if the radiation was waved in the general vicinity of my leg, the cancer could still survive. I loved the dogged determination of my physicians and gave an enthusiastic thumbs up when they told me they were going to "overkill my cancer."

I was about to embark on my own personal education of radiation. Everyone has heard about radiation, but what is it? According to the National Cancer Institute, radiation is beams of high energy waves or streams of particles. In high doses it can kill cancer cells or keep them from growing and dividing by damaging their genetic material. Cancer cells generally grow and divide faster than normal, healthy cells, so radiation is an effective treatment.

Normal cells are also affected but usually regenerate after the radiation treatments are complete. Of course, the idea is to radiate the unhealthy, cancer cells with minimal damage to any surrounding areas. Cancer cells do not regenerate unless you take a large amount of antioxidants during radiation. In this case, the cancer cells can repair themselves.

Radiation as an independent treatment source does not hurt and does not include the use of needles. According to Everydayhealth.com, side effects "include fatigue, skin irritation, temporary or permanent hair loss, temporary change in skin color in the treatment area, loss of appetite, nausea and vomiting, cramps, diarrhea," and a host of other things depending on your age, the state of your health at diagnosis, and the other medications or treatments you are taking simultaneously.

Radiation is conducted five days a week, followed by two days of much-needed recuperation. Each treatment only lasts a few minutes with x-rays taken once a week to ensure the radiation beams are being aimed in the right direction.

During radiation you lie down on a thin, padded table while an enormous piece of machinery starts rising toward the ceiling as it rotates around your body. The tech lines up the machine according to your tattoos and then leaves the room to turn on what sounds like a bug zapper for about sixty seconds. The tech then comes back into the room and rotates the machine underneath you. Another sixty-second zap and you are on your way out the door.

The piece of the machine that is rotating around your body is the size of the back half of my Suburban, and is brought into the room in smaller pieces and assembled inside. It is so precise that each year a group of physicists gather to disassemble it and make sure each piece is checked for accuracy before being reassembled and given a seal of approval for another twelve months.

Radiation is not only about daily hospital visits but also

the care you are receiving at home. Normally you can moisturize your skin with anything from forty-nine cent soap to designer caviar moisturizers. During radiation you have one moisturizing option—100 percent liquid aloe vera.

Why would your body crave moisture? As you continue to go through several weeks of treatments, the skin surrounding the affected area is usually dry and irritated, turning from a light reddish-pink color to a darker brown color. In children this color will normally fade, but often the brown tone stays in adults, as adult skin does not regenerate as quickly as younger, plumper skin does. My radiologist had warned me of darkening, cracking skin, so I was preparing myself for even more disgusting legs than I sported during my staph phase.

Healthy foods are a must during any kind of cancer treatment, but especially during radiation, to maintain your physical strength (almost an oxy moron). Eating foods high in calories and protein is a plus, though taking vitamins is not always recommended, and supplements may or may not be helpful. Of course, every person reacts differently to radiation, so that is why it is so important to meet with a physician on a regular basis while undergoing these treatments.

The long-term effects of radiation are minimal. Your body can feel tired and worn down for well over a year, and some report feelings of being totally overwhelmed by the exhaustion. I was already overwhelmed by the blessings and favor that were infused in every part of my treatment, and I was not about to give in to fear or exhaustion at this point.

I had educated myself on the facts regarding radiation, and now I was sitting in yet another waiting room, gearing up for my very first treatment. I was, by several decades, the youngest person there and the only one not eligible for retirement. I had no idea what to expect, and at the same time I expected only good things (Psalm 31:1–3).

The treatments each morning were lightning fast but took most of my energy for the remainder of the day. According to the National Cancer Institute, the fatigue caused during radiation treatments generally comes from stress, anemia, anxiety, depression, lack of activity, medicines, or any combination of the above. Most of the time you will not know why you are tired, just that you are. And the exhaustion increases with the length of the treatments.

My radiology technician was Cathy, and she would be with me every day for my five-week stint. She was absolutely precious, and just a joy to spend time with. She exuded the love for her job that was becoming commonplace at M.D. Anderson (Galatians 6:9–10).

The radiation rooms were in the basement, and Cathy escorted me into a wonderfully inviting room where Christian music was playing softly in the background. One of her friends who met me during my tattooing session told her I would probably enjoy her CD collection. She was right. I don't know what I had expected in a radiation lab, but this homey atmosphere was certainly not it.

The first time I lay down on the radiation table, the lyrics sang out loud and clear, "Do not be afraid. The problem that you're in is for My glory." I was completely at peace and knew that God was in complete control (Isaiah 40:31). As the light beams pierced my skin, I felt no pain or anxiety, only peace. Because of the intensity of the beams, I was not allowed to have my left leg lying next to the one being treated, so I held that leg next to my chest in order to keep the healthy tissue there from being destroyed. I looked like a flamingo lying under a bug zapper.

It was August 4, 2006, and the end of my first week of radiation. One down, four to go (Psalm 66:8–12). It was time for my first update with Dr. Ballo, who seemed extremely pleased to see my foot healing so nicely.

Amazingly enough, the radiation treatments weren't affecting my skin color in any way, which was shocking to both of us since my skin is so white it can glow in the dark. I get a sun burn on the way to the mailbox, so I was just waiting for the bottom half of my leg to look like a zebra.

With every passing day, I was growing more and more physically exhausted (Matthew 11:28–30). I thought I was tired when I brought my kids home from the hospital, but there were days during radiation that I wondered if anyone would notice if I slept through the entire weekend.

I continued reading Psalm 61 every day. I also loved Psalm 23. I was there. I was in the valley of the shadow of death. I could look around the hospital and see death in every hallway, sitting in every waiting room right next to me. I could almost taste death in the air that could easily have suffocated me.

But when I looked in the mirror every morning and saw the deep, dark creases under my eyes, I thanked God for giving me life. If it meant I only had one more day, I thanked him for giving me that very day (Psalm 27:13–14). I was one day closer to my healing.

I knew the severity of my disease, but I was not going to

let the disease conquer my spirit, my determination, or my resolve. Jesus had died on the cross many years before anyone thought about me, and he had conquered death, hell, and the grave. I took daily comfort in that—every morning when I had to literally drag myself out of bed to make my 9:00 a.m. radiation appointment. I am not a morning person by nature, so waking up is always a chore. However, waking up for radiation treatments was exceptionally challenging on many days.

If Jesus could endure the total and complete humiliation of the cross for someone like me, I could endure a little cancer without complaining. For this and many other reasons, I never asked God why I had cancer. It would be pointless.

Knowing that God is infinitely more intelligent than I, and obviously works off more than a five-year calendar, who was I to ask why? And if this was the direction my life was taking, then it was time to have faith that God would complete a good work within me (Philippians 1:6). I had failed him many times, but he had not failed me yet.

I thanked God every day for trusting me with this challenge and asked for strength to make it to the other side (Psalm 34). I didn't want the journey to be easier or shorter. I just wanted strength to run the race that had been set before me. I wanted to make it home to hold my kids one more time (Psalm 31:24). I wanted to see another birthday. I wanted to spend another Thanksgiving at the ranch and another Christmas at home under the tree with my family, listening to my husband complain when the dogs ate the ornaments and candy canes off the tree.

I was not going down without a fight. I was not a stranger to perseverance, but like so many other qualities, God was allowing me to hone this ability and reach him on a new level. He was allowing me to become stronger than ever, and he was using a terminal disease to drive home the message. I was listening intently.

During my daily visits to the hospital for radiation, it was not uncommon to see small children strapped to gurneys wheeled by teams of pediatric doctors on their way to treatment rooms. Here were these tiny human beings, unable to comprehend what was happening, undergoing the same treatments I was and in many cases enduring much more. These miniature patients were often too small to sit up on their own and had to be fastened into car seats or other devices to keep them from rolling off the hospital beds. Many of them had been fighting cancer their entire short lives.

Horrified parents were usually trailing closely behind, invariably donning a look of quiet desperation and helplessness on their faces. Any one of them would have taken the place of their child on that gurney without a moment's hesitation. It was a heart-wrenching spectacle. How would anyone have the grace to endure that?

During the seconds the babies were wheeled by with tubes coming from any body part large enough to support them, you could cut the silence with a knife. There were no words. I was grateful for the old men who shared my waiting room on a daily basis. They had already lived long, rich lives and had many wonderful memories, which they were constantly sharing with anyone within shouting distance. If I had a young mother with a tiny child sitting next to me every morning, the agony would be unbearable.

There were so many things to be thankful for with my own

cancer journey (Psalm 51:8–12). I was enormously grateful to be the one with cancer at my house, and not one of my children. As I watched these babies rushing through the hallways in every effort to extend their lives, I prayed that their healing would come soon and their parents' agony would find quick relief. Seeing sick children on TV makes you sad, but seeing them in living color breaks your heart. The drama is real and there are no commercial breaks. The reality is suffocating. It is a sight emblazoned on my memory forever.

By the end of my first week of radiation, I was an old pro.

I was there at M.D. Anderson for a reason, but only for a season. I was not growing roots, just passing the time with a smile on my face.

Let Mercy Rain

My husband was keeping my girls in San Antonio with the help of various family members and our fabulous nanny, Miss Amanda. Occasionally the kids would come to Houston and provide some much-needed comic relief. The girls were so full of life and limitless energy, the polar opposite of what I had been seeing every day. They were like rays of sunshine peeking through the clouds on a rainy day.

It was a welcome relief to be around tiny, healthy people who weren't undergoing major physical traumas or treatments and were not connected to any type of tubing. It was fantastic to be around people who didn't know I had a terminal disease and who didn't want to ask me about my leg. They just wanted to have fun and hang out with their mom (Psalm 95:1–3).

My parents have spent a lot of time and energy over the years teaching me right from wrong. It was my turn to teach my own children the same lessons, and I was grateful for the opportunity to show them how to rejoice by choice (Proverbs 22:6). Knowing they were too young to understand exactly what was going on was a huge relief for me. They didn't need to understand about laughing through the pain or that cancer kills. They loved Houston for the skating rink in the mall and knew Mommy was seeing a doctor for her broken leg. That was enough.

Each day brought a new wave of gratitude (Psalm 103:1–4). I was grateful for my children's health and that they were very young and naive. I was grateful to live in the United States where we take exceptional and immediate medical care for granted. The grace that was carrying me through this storm was also allowing me to forego the extra burden of sharing it with my children (Psalm 111:1).

My girls knew the doctors were trying to get the "germs" out of my body and, amazingly enough, would let the medical conversation end right there. Kassidee, three, and Mckenzie, five, would often wrap their legs in toilet paper and pretend to have a broken leg. One girl was the doctor and one was the patient. The "patient" would use one of my "crunches" (crutches) and hobble around, asking for medical attention.

When the week ended and the girls returned to San Antonio, the apartment in Houston would once again grow painfully silent. It would be too easy to give in to depression, so I immediately regained my focus and reminded myself of my mission (Psalm 86:1–7). I had to get well so that I could be a full-time mom once again. I would not be much help to my children from the graveyard.

Mckenzie and Kassidee were having the summer of their lives. Between visits to see me in Houston, they were at Disney World, the coast, staying with their cousins and grandparents, and generally enjoying a wonderful, fun-filled summer. I was elated that their attention was diverted from my not being home. This made it much easier for me to be gone.

One of the many wonderful things about prayer is that there is no distance where prayer cannot reach and no prayer too big for God to answer. If someone is praying for me in San Antonio or Israel, God still hears them interceding on my behalf. This was a continual source of comfort to me, as I knew many people were lifting me up when I was too exhausted to even think straight.

Each time someone reached out to me I felt as if God were kissing me on the forehead (Psalm 63:7). Every drop of God's goodness was like a new blessing, and I was soaking it all in. Ezekiel 34:26 says, "…and I will cause showers to come down in their season; there shall be showers of blessing."

I continued my daily radiation treatments, fully expecting my lily white skin to look like a dried-up lobster soon. After several more treatments, there was still no redness, save for the magic marker used to mark my radiation lines. In order to pinpoint the accuracy of the treatment, the technicians mark your leg in red, black, or blue markers to notate where the treatments need to take place. These are done in permanent markers that you cannot wash off. Most of the time my leg looked as if my three-year-old had used it for art class and tried turning it into an Easter egg.

Since I was taking radiation in the summer time, the markings were extremely attractive with my shorts. Yes, this lovely walking art gallery was fully visible to the viewing public at large. I loved going to the mall and watching people stare at my colorful legs as if I either hadn't noticed the vibrant coloration or forgot to bathe. When they stared just a little too long, I had lots of fun comments for them like, "I gave up bathing for lent," and "I'm practicing for my tattoo artistry final."

Life was good. There was no pain in my leg, and my doctor was pleased with my progress. My leg had beaten the odds and continued to heal. The skin had not cracked open as predicted and there was no oozing from the inside out, only healing. Dr. Ballo warned me that my treatments were going to be boring because everything was going so well. Since I am not a boring person, we both laughed and knew I would find a way to fill in the time.

One day while I was waiting for my radiation treatment, I noticed a young man in his forties sitting very close to me. My appointment was at 9:00 a.m. every morning, so I knew the normal crowd that hung out with me every day, knew their circumstances and had met their families. They had met mine.

This young man in his forties was a new face in the crowd. He held a plastic bowl in his lap in case he vomited while he was waiting. On the other side of this gentleman was another man awaiting his first round of radiation.

I could imagine what must be going through the new guy's mind as he was eyeing the other man's plastic barf bowl precariously sliding around on his lap. I went over to where he was sitting with his wife and explained how the radiation process worked, how fast the treatments are, and that the wait was the longest part of his day. I wanted to ease his apprehension and give him hope (John 15:11–12).

I explained to the couple how the man with the bowl was

taking more than radiation treatments. New guy thanked me for taking the time to explain the unknown to him, and I could visibly see the stress leaving the creases in his face (John 14:27). I smiled and said, "God bless you." Immediately his wife looked at me with tears in her eyes and said, "Thank you!"

I was having a great time in Houston, trying to make the most of my visit. It was like eating an elephant one bite at a time. I made friends with all of the doctors, nurses, hospital administration, book store volunteers, and coffee shop workers. Everyone smiled when they saw me coming. They knew God had filled me with joy and peace (John 16:33). In a hospital full of cancer patients, this was certainly unusual.

Emails continued to pour in, so I decided to start distributing a weekly email update on my treatments. Not everyone could figure out how to use the blog, so the email updates were an easy, user-friendly option.

The Bible says to pray specifically and cites the Lord's Prayer as our example (Matthew 6:9–13). I wanted the prayer warriors to know how to pray. I also wanted them to know that their prayers were working and to continue storming the gates of heaven on my behalf (Psalm 119:77).

My first email thanked everyone for their love, support, and prayers. I also shared a taste of what I had already learned during my brief stay at M.D. Anderson:

> God's mercy is vast, beyond our comprehension and deserving.
>
> I am thankful for the love demonstrated by people all over the world; not people who say "I love you," but people who are not afraid to put those words into action.

It is important to live today to the fullest, not put off thanking God until tomorrow for the time He has given us today.

Health is priceless.

I cannot afford to shop at the Galleria in Houston.

Work can wait.

My husband can run my household and pay the bills on time without my input or supervision.

Laughter is the best medicine, and it is absolutely free. No co-pay or consultation involved.

You are never too sick or tired to help the guy next to you. Helping someone else is greater than any treasure on earth.

You either get the cancer or the cancer gets you.

It is OK to accept help.

Life is very short; make your time count.

Most people don't know what to say when they find out you have a terminal disease. Offer a prayer or a smile, not advice, unless you have been there and bought the t-shirt.

Don't sweat the small stuff. Keep your eye on the prize.

Enjoy the people you love the most.

Be grateful for healthy, happy children.

As much as they would like to, parents can't fix everything.

Have the attitude of gratitude; it can save your life.

There is nothing in the past so great that it should be allowed to overshadow or control your future.

God's grace is sufficient.

By the end of the second week of radiation, I felt like I had aged ten years. I was ready to go home for the weekend. I missed my girls. I missed my husband. I missed my dogs. I wanted to sleep in my own bed and watch my own TV, even though I knew that meant I would be watching the Disney Channel.

I missed the sounds and smells of my own home. The kids were coming home from Disneyworld, and I knew they would be filled with wonderful fairy-tale stories about princesses and Mickey Mouse. I was ready for a fantasy injection. The rides I had been on most recently were not that fun and had no height requirements. The lines were way too long.

Another thing I missed was the sound of tiny (yet extremely loud) voices singing original compositions at all times of the day and night. My kids love to make up their own songs and dance around the living room while they sing into a pretend microphone. We enjoy singing together every day, because music can elevate you to a place where joy and worship abound (Psalm 86:12–13). As long as I was singing, I was filled with peace.

The Bible says that if we refuse to praise him, even the rocks will cry out (Luke 19:40). I didn't want to give the rocks a chance. I wanted God to know I was shouting his praise from the rafters (Psalm 138:1–3). I had been granted one more day to thank him for his mercy and grace in my life. That in itself was more than enough to shout about.

The weekend flew by in the blink of an eye, and it was time to leave Fantasy Island and head back to Houston and the harsh reality of Radiation Central.

A Mother's Guilt

It was the third week of radiation, and my daughter Mckenzie's sixth birthday. I had some kind of funky virus, strep throat, vomiting, nausea, and unrelenting exhaustion. My sickness only added to the physical stress of the treatments, and everyone at home was partyin' down and celebrating my daughter's birthday, complete with piñata, tons of family, and delicious food. I was missing it. I sat down on the floor in the center of my bedroom in our Houston apartment, remembering the day she was born, and cried.

I was blessed and elated to know my family was throwing a party for her in my absence, but I was crushed by my own guilt, knowing there was no way I could attend. I couldn't help Mckenzie pick out her favorite cake or watch her open gifts. She was old enough now to know what a birthday was, and I was miles away in an empty apartment. So I took a hot shower and put on my t-shirt that says "Cancer Sucks."

The following morning Mckenzie started kindergarten, and I cried all over again. This was an important week for her, and I was missing every bit of it. I was mad because I was crying. I was mad because I was so completely exhausted. I was mad to be stuck in a hospital in another city instead of somewhere closer to home.

I called Mckenzie during the opening ceremonies at school, and she sounded so excited to see her old friends again and to start a new school year. I was glad she wasn't missing me as much as I was missing her. My guilt was growing by the second.

Liz Barton, the elementary principal, called me to report that Mckenzie was doing fine in her new class. This single act of kindness greatly lifted my spirits; it made my heart smile. Unfortunately, the week dragged on as sickness and exhaustion consumed me. I was miserable.

My youngest daughter, Kassidee, was spending the week with me and my mother in Houston. Kassi had just turned four and was a bundle of non-stop energy who did not believe in naps. She always put a smile on my face with her great sense of humor and fantastically animated expressions. I wanted to bottle up her energy and drink it. When she leaned over to hug and kiss me, every problem in my world instantly dissolved (Psalm 127:3–4).

We read books together, watched videos, and played with Barbies on the couch. Kids respond to you. If you don't tell them it's a terrible week, they don't know. Kassi was happy to stay home and watch movies in bed with huge bowls of buttered popcorn and juice.

Houston was a vacation for her. She would make comments like, "I love our apartment in Houston, Mommy; it's really cool." I couldn't wait to leave it, and she was having the time of her life. It was a good lesson for me to just be content—to make the most of my circumstances, because there wasn't much I could do to change them (Hebrews 13:5).

Each morning, Kassidee woke up, dressed, and made the trek to the hospital with me. At the front desk we signed in per protocol, verifying that Kassi's shots were up to date. A painted name tag designed by one of the children receiving treatment from M.D. Anderson showed she was an approved guest for the day.

One morning as we checked in, Kassidee was given a sticker painted with a giant bright green frog on the front. Anxious to make idle chit chat to detract Kassi from our grim surroundings, I asked if she knew how to say frog in Spanish. She looked at me and scrunched her face, like, *You have got to be the dumbest person on earth to be asking me that*, and quickly responded, "Of course. It's ribbit, ribbit."

Kassi's presence was a constant reminder of why I was fighting so hard to live.

Another morning when we were dressing, she was looking through my jewelry in the bathroom drawer. Diana had given me a very special gold necklace with a cross on one side and "Fear not for I am with you" on the back. Kassi's favorite color of the month was gold, so it caught her attention immediately. She looked up at me with her huge blue eyes and said, "Mommy, Jesus died on that cross with his blood for you and for me." Sometimes it takes a little child to remind us of the true value of life (Mark 9:14–15).

By Friday, my third week of treatment was behind me, and my virus and strep were finally responding to antibiotics. I continued to thank God every day for his provision and his endless mercies (1 Chronicles 16:34). Being sick meant I was still part of the human race.

I wanted to be like the tea kettle, up to my neck in boiling water and singing loud and clear. At this point I probably sounded more like a drowned rat singing, but I was still singing (Psalm 33:3).

I started to surround myself with positive literature, inspirational sayings, Scripture verses, great song lyrics, and funny videos. I needed to feed my soul. My body was tired, but my spirit was still fighting. I refused to give up.

The third week of radiation was coming to a close, and it was time for another weekly email update:

Cancer brings a lot of clarity. The minutiae of life no longer matters. Neither do the little people that are constantly trying to bring you down. Life is just too short. The verse that I have read over and over since my treatments began is Psalm 61:1–4. "Hear my cry, O God; Attend to my prayer. From the end of the earth I will cry to You, When my heart is overwhelmed; Lead me to the rock that is higher than I. For you have been a shelter for me, A strong tower from the enemy. I will abide in Your tabernacle forever; I will trust in the shelter of Your wings."

It has been a good week because I am in the exact place that I need to be at the exact time. I am not too old to learn new lessons, and I am not too young to take them for granted. Fortunately, I'm smart enough to know that I don't know nearly enough.

My mom drove Kassidee and I home to San Antonio for the weekend so I could visit with Mckenzie and catch up on all of the exciting kindergarten news. She is a smart girl, and not much gets past her. Still, I was stunned when her big blue eyes looked up at me and said, "So, you only have two more weeks of radiation, huh?"

I was shocked she even knew the word radiation. I had never used that word in front of her, but I had been gone for a few weeks. Evidently her medical vocabulary had become more prolific in my absence.

I asked her what she knew about radiation. She said, "I know all about your treatment. The doctor comes in every day with his camera and takes a picture of your foot."

I smiled from ear to ear and asked, "How did you get to be so smart?" I laughed at the mental picture of my radiologist coming in with his Polaroid every day to photograph my leg. I would love for life to be that simple (2 Samuel 22:2–7, 33–34).

I started unpacking my suitcase and putting things back in my closet from my last two weeks in Houston. The junk in my suitcase seemed to have multiplied. I was trying to switch out my clothes and jewelry for the next two weeks when I ran across a silver ring Diana had brought back from Israel on a trip she had taken years before. It was a plain silver band with Hebrew writing on it. I had not seen the ring in years and could not remember what the inscription said. When I looked at the translation in the ring box, it read, "Fear not for I am with you even to the ends of the earth."

By the end of the weekend, Mckenzie and Kassidee were headed for the beach with my husband and the entire Hagee clan. I was laughing with them, talking about how much fun they would have on their trip with all of their cousins, and asking them to take lots of pictures on their Sponge Bob camera so they could tell me all about it. Kassidee had just spent the week with me, so she gladly waved goodbye as I walked toward my Suburban, headed to Houston for my fourth week of radiation.

Mckenzie should have been excited about getting an extra week of vacation away from school but instead began to sob uncontrollably, and I watched in horror as her tiny body shook from the force of her tears. She begged me to go to the beach with her and postpone my treatments for just one week.

"How many days will you be gone, Mommy?" Ten days. "How about just going for three days and then coming to the beach with us?" I began to suffocate once again from the crushing weight of a mother's guilt. But what were my options? I had to give her my best smile and quickly pack her, along with her toys, into the car headed for the beach before my knees gave out and my eyes flooded with tears.

Then it hit me. *What if all of this wonderful treatment doesn't work? What if the radiation doesn't shrink the tumor, and the cancer starts spreading? What if I die? Who will take care of my girls? Who will pay for their college tuition? Will they blame God for my death? Will they blame me for not fighting hard enough? Where will they live? Will the quality of their lives suffer? Who will put their hair in pigtails for school every day? How will I ever explain to them I have to leave forever, that they won't see me again until they get to heaven?*

I was not afraid to die. I knew where I was going. I was okay with that, but I did not want to leave my young, impressionable girls behind to be raised by someone else. Cancer was not something they would be able to comprehend for years to come. Mckenzie and Kassidee were pretending their legs were broken. But what if their hearts were irreparably broken? No amount of toilet paper in the world could fix that.

A mother's guilt can be overwhelming at times, and this was no exception. My mind was bombarded with what might happen to them if I died. I knew that living in Houston for the summer was the first step toward saving my life. Being away for a few weeks was no picnic, but it certainly beat being gone forever.

That night I got down on my knees once again (Isaiah 55:6). *God, if it is my time to go, then I am ready. I have had a great life filled with blessings beyond my deserving. I know that everyone is allotted a certain number of days, and if it is my time, then I am thankful for thirty-seven wonderful years. But if my death will in any way impact my children so that they will not grow up to serve you with their whole hearts, then please let me stick around just long enough to make sure they are on the right track. They have a rich Christian heritage, and I don't want them to miss out on the blessings that you have in store for them because I wasn't here to lead them down the right path. Don't let them lose their souls because I lost my life.*

I was temporarily down (physically) but certainly not out (Lamentations 3:22–26).

I didn't want to be bitter. I wanted to be better. I wanted to be exceptional. There was no honorable mention here, no silver medal. I had to win without apology. This was a winner takes all victory, and I was determined not to give an inch. The alternative was too grim.

I knew the Champion of Love had a plan in store for me that would knock my socks off. Of course, I hated to wait for the plan to unfold, but that's how God works. He is a God of the midnight hour who does not tell you anything ahead of time. Usually around 11:59:59 you find out the next step in the game of life, and if you are like me, you are holding your breath all the way to the finish line, trying to give God a little extra advice along the way.

I told God that what Satan meant for evil, I would use for good (Genesis 50:20). If Jesus gave his life for me, then it made sense he would give me enough time on earth to fulfill whatever purpose he had for me. I didn't think my mission was complete, and it was certainly not mission impossible. I was ready to bask in the shelter of his wings (Psalm 63:7–8).

If God gives you something it is a gift. Men give presents, but God gives gifts. When God gives you something, nothing and no one can take it away or destroy it unless you allow them to. John 16:33 says, "These things I have spoken to you, that in Me you may have peace. In the world you will have tribulation; but be of good cheer, I have overcome the world." If God had overcome the whole world, I could overcome a little cancer.

I was back in Houston, and we were off to the races as my fourth week of radiation began. I was crossing the days off on my calendar and had only ten treatments left before returning home for good. Reports were coming in from the coast that the girls were having a blast, and I felt the faint beginnings of my guilt subsiding. I was severely congested, and my hair was starting to break off, but I continued celebrating each day.

I was still surrounded by death on a daily basis. If you have a conscience, you cannot help but be affected by the startling reality and visual stimulus sent to your brain when you see a decaying body wheeled in front of you.

Just when you thought you had seen the end of the patient line, you realized it was just curving to the left and out of sight, wrapping around the building as a new set of patients was admitted. I prayed for the patients surrounding me every day in the treatment rooms and lobbies as I prayed for myself (2 Corinthians 1:3–5). None of us knew with any medical certainty exactly where we were headed.

I thought about what it would be like to be God. Talk about never catching a break. There are no vacation days in that line of work.

Since I was away from the office myself, but definitely not on vacation, I decided to make the most of my week as I was starting to feel much better. My uncle and cousin graciously hosted my mother and I for dinner, which was a welcome departure from hospital banter. It was great to be around healthy, humorous people and talk about non-cancer related things, to make jokes and laugh without people looking at you like you are being disrespectful.

The evening was a nice escape. In the restaurant, it was easy to forget the current complexity of my life while sipping on sweet ice tea with ice cubes clinking the glass. I soaked in every delicious moment, relishing the fact that everyone around me was healthy and could get to the car without the aide of a wheelchair or cane, without an oxygen mask or IVs attached. But all good things must come to an end, and in short order I was headed back to my apartment for a few hours of sleep before my next round of treatment and tests began.

This new round of tests that I had just completed the day

before showed that my chest x-rays were clear. The cancer still hadn't spread, thank God. Since my cancer was labeled as very aggressive, the doctors were constantly checking to see if the cancer had moved up my leg and into my lungs.

A quick fact about cancer is that, if you have breast cancer and it moves to another part of your body (for example, your leg), it is still considered breast cancer. Since I had been diagnosed with leiomyosarcoma, no matter where it moved, it would still be this same kind of cancer. Of course, you can develop a second type of cancer in another area of your body, but this is very unusual.

My x-rays had just come back clean as a whistle, and this was an enormous reason for celebration, a promise that God was not yet finished with me. I was not going to be a statistic (Jeremiah 32:17).

Dr. Cannon was the new oncologist assigned to my case, as my previous oncologist was moving to another hospital to open his own sarcoma wing. M.D. Anderson is a teaching hospital that allows doctors to hone their skills and practice for several years while teaching others. Oftentimes these doctors are offered their own hospital wings or various practices around the country, as they are the best and brightest in their fields.

M.D. Anderson is also a hospital that is second to none in cutting-edge research and modern technology. I was with the best of the best, and it felt great to be part of a team that was not satisfied with mediocrity!

I was still undergoing radiation, but it was time to head over to the Sarcoma Center once again to meet my new oncologist face-to-face. As I waited for my first appointment with Dr. Cannon, I watched a young man with jet black hair and pale white skin about my age sitting in a wheelchair. He was holding the side of his face and wincing as he quietly sobbed from the excruciating pain. His dad looked directly at me with enormous, sad brown eyes that pierced my soul. It was as if one parent was telling another that their worst nightmare had been realized. A parent who can exercise every privilege in their power and not make a difference in their child's life or death situation is truly a parent whose heart is breaking into millions of shards just one tiny piece at a time.

There was nothing this father could do to help his son. The father's countenance registered a great sense of silent desperation and overwhelming sadness tempered with guilt. I have no doubt that he would have given everything that he owned to take his son's pain away, or to trade places with him, yet he could do nothing to relieve or even lessen the pain for sixty seconds.

I will never forget the look in that father's dark and brooding eyes as his son joined the ranks of so many searching for a cure to their particular brand of cancer. He reminded me of a man feverishly treading water in a shark-infested ocean, searching for a rescue boat. To this day I wonder if the father's heartache was greater than the son's physical pain. Surely there is no greater sadness in life than to know you cannot help your child.

I remembered Peter when he was standing on the sea shore and saw Jesus standing in the bow of the boat. Peter called out to Jesus and started walking on the water (Matthew 14:26–36). As long as Peter remained focused on the Lord, he had no problem. There was no need for a life jacket. When Peter looked at his surroundings, he quickly began to sink.

Cancer was my ocean, an ocean I shared with countless millions. I did not want this unforgiving and tumultuous ocean to swallow me whole. I wanted to maintain such an intense focus on God's Word that I could quickly and easily walk across the water and jump in the boat. I wanted to get off the cancer cruise, and I was willing to endure whatever terms God dictated in order to fit his perfect will for my life. Every day that I opened my eyes, I was a living miracle, beating overwhelming odds.

My mental picture of Peter walking on the water dissipated quickly when my name was called. It was my turn to meet Dr. Cannon. I thought I had prepared myself for whatever news came my way at this point. I mean, how much more shocking can the news be than a cancer diagnosis over the phone?

Today's news included the fun fact that I would need a second surgery. This was not totally unexpected, so it didn't send me over the edge (Psalm 138:7–8). After all, if there were any cancer cells still living in my ankle, I wanted someone to cut them out pronto. Why put off for tomorrow what you can cut out today? Originally Dr. Yasko thought this might not be necessary, but the doctors were now certain that some cancer cells were more than likely left behind after the original excision, so they wanted to go in and clean out the entire area.

For this second surgery, the doctors would make a deep incision into the original surgical site and remove all of the connective tissues, small muscles, and blood vessels down to the bone. This was the area most likely affected with the highest potential of spreading any cancer up my leg or to my chest.

The doctors were not going to remove my foot or any bones and planned on reconstructing my lower leg using parts generously donated by my upper leg. No rods, pins, or foreign objects would be placed in my leg. One of my inner thigh muscles (grisailles) would be reattached at my ankle, including the blood vessels and surrounding tissue. My outer thigh would donate skin to cover the muscle.

I started asking my fabulous plastic surgeon, Dr. Oatesates, to please use some of the extra fat in my thigh around the muscle and skin grafts for the reconstruction. He was laughing. I was serious. I told him I was the only woman ever to go to a plastic surgeon and come out with a fatter leg. But I still had my leg (Psalm 139:14–16). If God had brought me this far, he was not going to let me down now (Psalm 111:1–4, 10).

Initially I was told that this re-constructive surgery would take anywhere from six to eight hours to complete and my leg would need at least six months to heal. It would be at least a year before further adjustments could be made to reshape the leg after the muscle and cells adapted to their new location in my body and became fully functional as if they were originally formed in that region of my body.

My team of doctors decided that I needed to complete my last few weeks of radiation and give my body at least a month without treatments of any kind in order to recover before the second surgery would be scheduled. I had no idea why we needed to wait between the radiation and the surgery. As far as I was concerned, the sooner my body was rid of any remaining cancer cells, the better.

I had no idea how completely worn out my body would be from the radiation, but as I closed in on the fifth and final week of my treatment, the stark realization of complete exhaustion hit me like Ben Franklin with his kite. I was so tired you could have knocked me over with a feather. My heart and soul were ready to go full steam ahead, but my body demanded a break. My hair continued to break off, and my face broke out, but I was emotionally and spiritually ready for the surgery because it was the next thing on my checklist that got me one step closer to God's promise of total healing.

God had already been carrying me through the storm (Malachi 4:2). Facing another, more monumental surgery that the doctors were calling "a big deal," I called in the "big guns" once again. I started contacting my prayer warriors to surround me with prayer and fasting so that this would be my last and final fight in the ring with cancer. My gloves were on, and all I needed was faith the size of a mustard seed for God to move heaven and earth just for me (Matthew 17:20–21).

I knew what we consider seemingly insurmountable or impossible barely registered as a challenge for God. What I was up against was a piece of cake for the Almighty, so I began to thank God all over again that I was keeping my leg. I would be able to walk again after some time and physical therapy.

During the surgery, the oncologist would be the first up at bat, as he cut away all muscle and tissue down to the bone. These small slivers of tissue would then be sent immediately to a pathologist to study under the microscope to ensure all of the cancer cells were cut out and only clean healthy cells remained. This process of slicing and dicing would continue until the pathologist verified there were no more cancer cells showing up on the slices under his microscope. At the onset of the surgery, no one knew exactly how much of my leg would have to be cut out.

The plastic surgeon would reconstruct my right leg based

on the amount of tissue removed by the oncologist. After determining how much of my upper thigh was needed to fill in the gap left in my lower leg, the plastic surgeon would begin cutting on the inside of my thigh, removing muscles, tissue, and blood vessels. Much to my chagrin, he would not remove any fatty tissue.

The blood vessels would then be painstakingly stitched in under a microscope to maintain perfect blood flow. If the vessels collapsed or didn't function properly, the plastic surgeon would have to search for another vessel in my leg and start the procedure over. After all of the tissue, muscle, and vessels were re-attached into the cavity left in my lower leg and ankle, the skin flap from the outside of my right thigh would be cut out and stitched over the entire donor site. It was a massive undertaking with multiple layers painstakingly stitched precisely into place, and I was planning on sleeping through the entire thing.

After visiting with Dr. Cannon, I had a basic plan of where I would be headed in two weeks after my radiation was complete. It was Wednesday, so this meant my next stop was Dr. Ballo's office, my radiologist, for my fourth consultation with him regarding my progress. I was sad that I wouldn't be seeing much of him anymore but elated to have radiation behind me. I was finally starting to see some light at the end of my tunnel and happy to know it was not a freight train after all.

When I first met Dr. Ballo, he was very concerned about the staph infection in my leg. Over the past month, we both witnessed miraculous healing taking place in that same leg right before our eyes. No one expected me to heal so quickly or so completely during this aggravating and exhausting process. I was almost finished with my radiation treatments, and there was barely a color change in my ankle. The faint lines showing where the radiation had been taking place made my radiologist happy. He was glad to see that the treatment was effective but not destroying my skin.

Matthew 8:27 says, "Who can this be, that even the winds and the sea obey Him?" I knew without a shadow of a doubt that when I had asked my prayer warriors to get down on their knees, God had taken charge of every affected cell in my body, and the physical storm that was raging within was just waiting to be calmed.

After spending several weeks with my wonderfully humorous and brilliant radiologist, we had become friends. I would miss his sense of humor when I no longer needed the radiation treatments, so I looked for as many reasons as I could find for us to laugh together before our final consultation.

I showed up for my next to last appointment wearing bright pink sandals dripping with large faux gemstones. Since I hadn't been able to wear any non-orthopedic shoes for a while, I was making up for lost time—fat, nasty foot and all. When Dr. Ballo saw my shoes, he grinned from ear to ear and said, "I'm glad to see you are wearing sensible shoes." We both laughed out loud as I walked out the door. I will forever be grateful to Dr. Ballo for his life-saving help and friendly demeanor during this most challenging time.

The rest of the week was uneventful, and it was once again time for my weekly email update:

This week I spent several hours at MD Anderson undergoing treatments, x-rays, tests and evaluations. I waited for hours that sometimes seemed like days. I think about how ironic it is that God would allow me to have a disease that makes you wait and wait and wait, and gives you only temporary results. I hate waiting. Doesn't everyone yell at the microwave to hurry up? I am now faced with a disease where time is a precious commodity, and I am forced to wait to find out just how much time I have. Irony.

I think about the irony of our society. We are all so busy trying to make our lives better that we don't realize how great our lives already are. We are too busy stepping on the roses to smell them. We only slow down when the thorns of life scratch us.

I don't know why God is merciful, but I am glad that he is. People often ask me, "Why did this happen to you? You are a good person." I tell them, "Why not me?" Had I not had this very rare and aggressive disease I would not have the firsthand knowledge of God's unmerited mercy and grace.

Because of your prayers, God has given me a second chance at life. I will never again take that for granted. Blessings to you all for standing with me during this time.

Shut Up and Pray!

Several weeks of radiation had taken me to a new level of physical exhaustion I had never known existed. This was certainly not the Land of Milk and Honey, but I was not complaining. I was grateful for world-class physicians that practiced cutting-edge medicine just a few hours down the road, practically in my backyard. And with the promise of each new day, God continued to remind me that he had not forgotten about my circumstances. He was not too busy to hear me like I had previously been when he had called upon me (Isaiah 35: 3–6).

One thing I kept hearing again and again that irritated me to the core was the phrase, "I know how you feel." I wanted to scream. No one knew exactly how I felt. Even if they were in the same boat, they could not possibly know *exactly* how I felt. Cancer affects everyone differently.

Just like you can't tell a pregnant woman you know exactly how the birth of her baby is going to go or that she looks fantastic now that she's gained one hundred pounds and has to wear a mumu. Pregnancy and cancer are emotional times.

When in doubt, do without giving your unsolicited advice

and avoid repeating the story of the last guy you know who died from the disease. Do without crushing the last bit of hope that person is clinging to. Just smile, offer to keep them in your prayers, and move on. Remember your mother's advice, "If you don't have something nice to say, don't say anything at all."

The truth is that we are all armchair quarterbacks. We can all solve everyone else's problems, but we are often blind to our own (Matthew 7:3–4). When someone tells you they are going through devastating circumstances, the last thing you need to say is, "I know exactly how you feel." Try saying something like, "I can only imagine what you must be going through, and please know that I will be praying for you. God knows exactly what you need."

The greatest gift you can give someone is love (John 15:12). Love someone enough to pray for them (Leviticus 19:18). How would you feel if you were in this same situation? If it was your spouse, child, mother, father, sister, brother? Would you spend time telling them how hopeless their situation is, talking about statistics, or would you want to do everything in your power to help them? Cancer patients know the odds are stacked against them. They do not need to be reminded.

Stop giving advice on things you know nothing about. If you can't tell someone you will pray for them in faith, believing for their complete healing, just shut up. Sometimes it is the greatest blessing when someone stops talking.

Generally in situations that involve death, dying, or decay, people have no idea what to say or how to appropriately express their sympathy. Most people enjoy hearing their own voice, so they make something up that they feel is some fantastic psychological or philosophical gem that the world cannot continue rotating on its axis without. That is not consoling. Just say you will put their needs before Jehovah God and walk away. If you are not a licensed professional, people are not as impressed with your ideas as your mother was.

I had heard my fill of unsolicited opinions with no medical backing at all as I began my fifth and final week of radiation. I had a spring in my limp and was looking forward to crossing the finish line. I was just a few short days away from reuniting with my family and celebrating the amazing things that God was doing in my life (Psalm 150). I was genuinely looking forward to going home and sleeping in my own bed then waking up to feed my deer in the front yard by hand. I was more than ready to see the Alamo City and trade the Galleria for my old familiar Target down the street.

My motto for the week was, "We are only as rich or as poor as we choose to be." I was not referring to money. Wealth can be measured in many ways other than finances. I wasn't going to wait until my treatments were over to begin living again. I wanted to enjoy whatever time was delegated to me, living life to the fullest. I told anybody that would sit still long enough how God had carried me through the toughest storm of my life and I had walked on water (Proverbs 3:5–8, 24–26).

Of course, Satan continued to remind me of the vast ocean that surrounded me, and I could once again hear the theme song to Jaws playing in the silent background. This week kicked off with another stiff shot of reality. Moved to another waiting area while my radiation machine was being repaired, I was once again the youngest member of the old man's club.

In between complaints, the old guys who shared in my daily wait for radiation treatments during that final week traded stories about the "good old days" to pass the time. Some days they would sit around and try to outdo one another with their fantastic tales of days gone by. As sad as it was to watch these sweet men in their golden years spending time in a hospital, it was somehow easier to digest than watching the infants pass by on gurneys.

Just as this thought popped into my mind, there it came—another tiny person on their way to treatment with needles and IVs hanging off every available limb. There was a baby blanket swallowing the tiny figure that was completely shrouded underneath and covered in medical equipment. A leg the size and color of a small porcelain doll poked out from underneath to tell a horrific story that no one wanted to be witness to.

This gurney held someone's precious baby girl who had been born with cancer. Not one disease-free day. Her tiny bald head pushed its way out of the blanket to reveal a pair of eyes that lacked the necessary understanding to process the treatment for such a grave and heartless disease. Where was she going, and would she survive? This precious angel could not have been more than a few months old. I was totally heartbroken for the mother, sad that her child may never see adulthood, glad that it was not my own child, guilty for being glad my children were healthy at home, and grateful that my cancer was currently being contained all in the same instant.

The morbid sight of a young life zapped of health at birth is something that completely robs you of breath and fills every empty space in your body with deep sorrow. I was inexplicably sad for the parents holding onto the gurney as it passed and the weight they must be carrying, knowing they would be questioning if they could have done anything differently to bypass this cancer from the very onset of their child's life.

I would never wish this disease on anyone, but at that moment I was most grateful that if someone in my family was infected it was me. My children and family members were at home, happy and healthy. I prayed that this tiny angel would be allowed to return home, happy, healthy, and whole.

Psalm 34: 17–20 says, "The righteous cry out, and the Lord hears, and delivers them out of all their troubles. The Lord is near to those who have a broken heart, and saves such as have a contrite spirit. Many are the afflictions of the righteous, but the Lord delivers him from them all. He guards all of his bones; not one of them is broken." I knew the Lord must be very close to the mother of this baby.

It is ironic what parenthood does for you. I was suffocating from guilt having to be away from my own children for much of the summer. The mother passing by with her child on the gurney would have traded places with me in a flash. She was drowning in guilt because she was at the hospital *with* her child.

It doesn't matter if you have cancer yourself or if it is your family member who is affected by the disease. A terminal disease affects every member of your family. It is a drenching sadness that rains on everyone's parade, the pink elephant in the room that everyone wants to know about but no one really wants to ask.

Life goes on back at home while you are away at the hospital, but it is not business as usual. There is a somberness that coats the atmosphere like the relentless humidity of a Texas summer (Psalm 42:11). If you have people close to you who will support you through prayer and fasting, you are truly blessed.

I wanted to make one final trip to the Houston Galleria before leaving town, to reward my youngest daughter, Kassidee, for enduring several less than thrilling days with me. The first stop on our trek was the Build-A-Bear Workshop, an endless row of various stuffed animals and more accessories than your vacuum can possibly suck up in one afternoon. But this was her request, and it was time for me to make good on my promise (Psalm 127:3–5).

It was a fun diversion for both of us from the land of unrelenting reality we had recently been immersed in. While Kassi was debating between a brown, blue, or white bear and a spotted, stuffed cheetah, one of the workers stopped me and pointed to my leg.

"Do you mind if I ask you if you have a staph infection?" I really wanted to slap her and ask if the store required IQ tests for employment. Instead I smiled and said, "No, actually I had a cancerous tumor removed, and I'm here for treatment at M.D. Anderson."

Obviously she didn't appreciate the sarcasm in my tone because she continued with, "Well, that's good because staph is really disgusting." And since I am usually not at a loss for comebacks, I smiled and said, "I am certainly glad that my cancer doesn't offend you." What an idiot! What person in their right mind would choose to have cancer over a staph infection so as not to offend a mall worker?

I don't think people truly understand how toxic their tongues can be. My five-year-old would say, "Zip it. Lock it. And put it in your pocket."

The Bell of Redemption

It was time for my final meeting with Dr. Ballo, my radiologist. His warm smile lit up the room as I thanked him for helping me. The doctor who had entered my life with staunch sobriety was now stopping to chat with me in the Starbucks line at M.D. Anderson and commenting on my bling-bling shoes. He found me with a grossly infected leg and left me with a heart full of hope.

Dr. Ballo gladly reported he would not see me again for treatment because my prognosis was very, very good. I was elated at hearing that phrase attached to my health once again. I had not heard that in a long time. I was deeply moved by Dr. Ballo's sincere dedication to a job he obviously loved. How can you truly thank someone for helping to save your life? It seemed a futile effort.

The night before my last radiation treatment, we were invited to dinner at the home of Joan and Stanford Alexander, an extremely sweet couple who was introduced to us by the

Leibmans. Both Mr. and Mrs. Alexander are cancer survivors and very active at M.D. Anderson. Mr. Alexander was the previous president of MDA and served on the board.

During our first week in Houston, the Alexanders arranged a meeting for me with Dr. Mendelsohn, the CEO of M.D. Anderson. I'm sure he had a few other things on his plate that week, but he greeted me warmly with an outstretched hand and made me feel welcome upon entering his private office at the hospital.

I went to dinner at the Alexanders' fully expecting to thank them for all they had done for me and for their many kindnesses. Again, words were a weak tribute to a family who had done so much to help me before we had even met. I wanted to express my sincere gratitude for their role in the phenomenal and very personalized treatment I had received since arriving at M.D. Anderson.

The staff and medical personnel had all gone above and beyond the call of duty to assist me in every way, treating me like a family member, not a number. Before I could utter a word of thanks, Mr. Alexander began telling me that Dr. Mendelsohn had just told him that week how complimentary all of the staff had been about me, how much they enjoyed working with me.

These were two men running major corporations having a conversation about *me*. I was exceptionally honored and humbled at the same time. God was letting me know for the one millionth time that he was right there with me, showing me undeserved mercy and favor. What a wonderful evening we shared, visiting with precious people. The Alexanders are angels here on earth, and they had reached out to help me, someone who before that evening was a complete stranger.

Friday, September 1, 2006, was my much-anticipated last day of radiation. It was certainly a red letter day in my life. I was dancing on the ceiling. When I arrived each morning for treatment that final week, Cathy, my radiology technician, counted down the days for me and acted as if she were my own personal cheerleader, supporting me all the way to the finish line. She was incredibly supportive and helpful throughout the five weeks of radiology, and by the end I felt like I was leaving a friend behind.

After my final treatment, Cathy gave me a beautiful card I will forever treasure. It was another bitter sweet ending. I was over the moon to have finished radiation but sad to leave Cathy. We'd traded kid stories every day, and she had become a bright and shining star while I trudged through a very dark valley.

When Dr. Ballo first told me I was going to be spending five weeks in Houston and coming into the hospital five days a week for radiation, it seemed like an ominous eternity. I did not know how I would live in another city, not working, away from my family, not doing anything but going to the hospital every day, and not go crazy. Now it was over with the blink of an eye. I was finished and filled to the rim with the absolute joy that only comes with certain triumph (James 1:2).

My treatments were over, and Kassidee was with me as Cathy led us down the hall toward a maritime bell displayed on the wall. Several years ago a naval officer donated a ship's bell after receiving his own treatment. Today, when someone finishes radiation, they get to ring the bell loud and clear so that anyone within hearing distance can join in the celebration.

There are congratulations all around. Every nurse, every

patient, every one with a voice is shouting for joy. There are no moments of silence here. There is much to be thankful for when you reach your last day of radiation. You are alive, and your cancer is shrinking. It is an enormous sense of accomplishment like none other.

As Kassidee and I stood in the hospital hallway and looked at this huge bell, hot tears of gratitude poured down my face as the bell began to clang loudly for all to hear. It was singing a song of my salvation and healing. It was singing a song of re-birth. I didn't want the clanging to stop. I wanted everyone to know that I had lived to tell about limitless mercy and unfailing grace. I made it.

I was grateful for modern medicine and that my treatments had gone so smoothly. I was grateful the cancer hadn't spread. I was grateful that my three-year-old daughter who had gone to so many treatments with me had absolutely no idea why I was really there. Most of all I was grateful for a Savior who died on a tree for me so long ago, so that I might live (Hebrews 12:2).

I was also grateful for God's love. How could he love me so much that he would send his only Son to die for *me*? He held the balance of the universe in the palm of his hand. I had disappointed him so many times, yet when I truly needed him, he was there for me. He didn't tell me he was too busy or that he would get back with me as soon as he helped a few million other people.

He came to help me in my very darkest hour and was not one second late. And because Jesus, the only perfect person who ever lived on this earth, went to the cross and died in my place, I was standing there victoriously ringing a bell in a cancer ward (1 Peter 1:3–7).

The stream of joy racing through my mind at this point far outweighed any amount of questions that had previously infiltrated every pore of my being upon my cancer diagnosis.

Thank you, God! Thank you for saving me. Thank you for dying in my place so that today I can stand next to my tiny daughter who has no idea what I'm really celebrating. Thank you that my life is not yet over. Thank you for not being finished with me yet. Thank you for not giving up on me. Thank you for putting me in the right place, with the right medical teams at the right time. Thank you for this treatment. Thank you for your unmerited mercy and love. Thank you for standing with me in the middle of this very hot fire. Thank you for reaching all the way down to Houston, Texas, to save a sinner like me. Thank you so much! I don't know how and I surely don't know why, but thank you!

That day was like a second birth-day for me. I was being given a second chance at life, and no one could really explain why. No doctor could tell me how or when I contracted this disease, and no one expected my treatments to go so smoothly. Now my treatments were over. It was a great day!

My last email was sent from my apartment before leaving Houston.

Cancer teaches you many things like how to roll with the punches. You learn that best laid plans mean nothing. Tomorrow you might be too sick to think … if you are fortunate enough to see tomorrow. Gratitude is taken to another level. There is always someone that has a heavier cross to bear. Looking around the treatment areas, I wonder why we spend countless hours pondering our outward appearance, when it is our interior we should be most concerned about. I also learned that I cannot last all day at the mall like I used to. I guess God has finally answered my husband's prayers.

This has been a golden opportunity for me to pull from my inner strength and reach out to a crowd I never thought I would belong to, the cancer club. It still sounds strange to say that I have cancer, but it is the current reality of my life. What have you survived, and who has benefited from your experience?

Today I took my last radiation treatment. When I finished, I rang the bell in the hallway of M.D. Anderson, letting everyone know I had my very last treatment. In a way, it will be another type of salvation for me. As I have seen in these hallways firsthand, everyone has a story. I am so grateful that no matter what happens to my body, my story will have a happy ending. God is so good!

It was time for me to move out of the apartment in Houston and head for home sweet home in San Antonio. This time my visit would not just be for the weekend. Victory never smelled so sweet! I was thrilled with the anticipation of being stuck in a Suburban piled high with my junk that had accumulated over the summer and listening to my three-year-old daughter ask a million exhausting questions about anything that popped into her young mind.

Radiation was over. Before the end of the day, I would have both of my precious girls on my lap with popcorn and Cokes, snuggled in my own bed, watching my own TV, with my dogs nearby wagging their tails from the excitement of my return. It was definitely a day worthy of much celebration!

I was so elated to have completed my radiation treatments that I wanted the newscasters to announce it on the red ticker tape that runs along the bottom of the CNN News screen. I wanted the local news to carry a true human interest story of

God's healing power. It was a newsworthy day in my life, and I wanted the world to know about it (Daniel 4:2–3).

God's mercy and grace were not lost on me. I knew he was ever present. Just in case I needed a reminder while I was away from home, there was a friend, relative, or complete stranger who would call, email, send a package, mail a card, or come by my treatment area to let me know they were praying for me. I lacked for nothing in a place of great need (Habakkuk 3:17–19).

I packed my stuff as if the apartment building were on fire. I didn't care if my shoes were in with the DVDs or if shampoo was dripping on my t-shirts. I wanted to get out of there. I was ready to be home. Home truly is where the heart is, and it was a luxury I had previously not appreciated as much as I did the day my radiation ended. I continued packing up boxes and boxes of anything in my path, as I was quite certain I could almost sprint all the way from Houston to San Antonio.

We needed some help loading the bigger boxes into the back of the Suburban, so we hired a kind man who turned out to be a cancer survivor to help us load the boxes that had hurriedly been thrown together. He had been walking by our apartment while we were preparing to leave, and we asked if he would mind helping us load a few things in the car. I'm sure if he would have seen the number of boxes we had, he would have changed his mind. Who in their right mind volunteers to help anyone move during a Texas summer?

What were the odds that he was a cancer survivor on this most triumphant day? His treatments were completed a few years earlier, but he still had some rough days now and then. He told me, "*A veces es mucho pelear la guerra, pero todavía estoy bailando.*" In English this translates, "Sometimes it's a lot to fight the battle, but I am still dancing." What a perfect gift on my way out of town.

The drive flew by, and once again I was pulling into my driveway. I was home for good. My oldest daughter, who had remained in San Antonio for school, was jumping up and down on the front porch, waving her arms in the air when she saw me walking up the driveway with suitcase in tow. Yes, it was a day of celebration for many from start to finish!

The following week it was time to get back to the reality of a full-time bank job while fighting residual fatigue from radiation. I work as a home loan officer, so the more I work, the more loans I close. The more loans I close, the more I get paid. I knew the bills from my recent hospital stay would be in my mailbox very soon, so I needed to get back on top of my game.

I was determined to work as efficiently as possible, as I only had a few short weeks before heading back to Houston for my second surgery. I was not anxious or overly concerned about the surgery but wondered how I was going to get any loans closed during this tiny window of opportunity.

I knew the pending surgery would include an intense and lengthy recovery, so time was of the essence at the office. I needed to get new loans on the system, clean my house, move our fall clothes in from the garage to prepare for a change in seasons, bathe my dogs, take extra toys to the daycare, and catch up with all mail and correspondence that my husband had accumulated at home during my absence. I also needed to make sure the girls had adequate school supplies, shoes, and clothes. Normally this would not have been a huge chore, but my body was worn out, and these menial tasks turned into a monumental and draining undertaking.

Once again, God sent an unexpected but most welcome answer. Mark, one of my co-workers, helped me complete loan applications and meet deadlines for my customers during my radiation treatments when I was trying to work from the condo in Houston. Obviously a glutton for punishment, Mark told me he would follow up on all of my loans while I was in the hospital so that my closings took place on time.

I explained that the complexity of the surgery would mandate my absence from the office for an extended period of time. Mark didn't care. He asked me what I was working on and graciously volunteered to take care of everything while I was out of the office.

My "to do" list was growing longer by the minute. Now that people knew I was home again and announcements were made that a second surgery was imminent, the "friendly" Christians started calling. "Aren't you afraid of what might happen during your surgery?" "When will they be cutting your leg off?"

There was not a frightened cell in my body, but several cells were becoming seriously annoyed. If the Scripture told us 365 times to "fear not," that was enough for me. I assumed anyone with two brain cells rubbing together could figure it out, but there is an old saying about assuming.

My phone was melting off the wall. One lady came over to pray for me with a group of my friends and literally five seconds later asked me, "So, they really are going to cut your leg off after all of this is over, right?" I looked at her and said, "Did you miss the part about the doctors saying there would be no amputation? Perhaps the 'very, very good prognosis' from my radiologist wasn't clear enough for you. Hold on, and I will repeat that slowly so you can better understand."

The spirit of slap came over me, and I had to stop myself from drawing a chart so that even Ellie Mae could understand what I was saying. Obviously she wasn't getting the big picture, and at this point in my ballgame I had to be surrounded with people who absolutely believed in the success of my upcoming surgery. There was no room for doubt here.

The Bible says to pray without ceasing and to pray in faith believing that God will give you the desires of your heart (1 Thessalonians 5:16–18). Healing was the absolute desire of my heart, and I knew that this was not out of the realm of his capabilities.

Most of what we are afraid of never happens. Much of the bad that happens in our lives is a result of our own poor choices, whether we want to admit it or not. I have not always made spectacular choices in my life, but I knew that going into a comprehensive surgery to save my life was a good choice, if not an optional one. I was still a little bummed that my plastic surgeon didn't want to donate the extra fat cells on my leg to science, but I was mentally prepared for this life-saving surgery.

I knew thousands of people were praying and fasting for me on a daily basis across the country, and I knew that Mark could easily handle my workload while I was away from the office. I was 100 percent sure that the surgery would be just another success story in the long line of great favor he had already shown me. I was also certain that God was leaning down from heaven with his hand cupped around his ear, listening to the prayers of his people who were crying out on my behalf (Colossians 4:2).

God knew the number of radiated and fried hairs on my head (Matthew 10:30–31). He had already taken care of my surgery before it ever happened (Psalm 139). It was a done deal before I was even born (Philippians 4:19–20).

What a Difference
a Day Makes

During the time between radiation and my second surgery, I made a quick daytrip to Houston to meet with my plastic surgeon. I love Dr. Oates. What a wonderfully humorous and kind man to be around!

Dr. Oates is brilliant but extremely humble, and always puts a huge smile on my face. He explained again what would take place the day of my surgery, and I reminded him to please take off any fat cells he ran across during the procedure. He smiled, and I knew it was a lost cause, but you can't blame a girl for trying.

The surgery sounded easy enough to me. I was going to be napping the whole time under deep sedation, so I was fine with whatever they wanted to carve out. Cut away! I told Dr. Oates that I didn't want to be like one of those horror movies where the patient wakes up halfway through the surgery while the doctor is still cutting. His warm laughter floated through the air as he assured me that wasn't going to happen.

I understood the gravity of this surgery, but it was a life-saving effort, so there was no reason to question or worry about it. I worry about the things I can change, but there are some things you must accept at face value (Matthew 6:25–34). This surgery was just one of those things. The joy of the Lord was my strength, for it makes rich and adds no sorrow (James 1:2). It was the next step in my journey, another checkmark on my list. I was ready.

Dr. Oates went on to explain that Dr. Cannon would begin the surgery, and then he would clean up the mess and refill the gap left behind by the oncologist. It was a massive and delicate undertaking that I would not completely appreciate until long after the surgery was performed.

I had horrendous and grotesque images of a gigantic and misshapen, elephant leg coming home with me, but it would still be *my* leg with no foreign parts or metal pins. I would not be setting off alarms at the airport. The doctors weren't cutting off my leg or cutting out any bones. The disease hadn't spread to my blood stream or affected my lungs or penetrated the bones. The laundry list of things to be grateful for was growing by leaps and bounds as I continued running non-stop errands in preparation for the big day.

The time spent at home with family and friends flew by. There were not enough hours in the day. On Monday, October 16, 2006, I went back to M.D. Anderson for one final round of testing before surgery. Psalm 118:17 says, "I will not die, but live and declare the works of the Lord." I had quoted this verse many times before, and this week it became my motto—literally words to live by.

As I ate dinner in Houston at our favorite Italian restaurant with Dad, Diana, and Jim, the night before my marathon surgery, the tension and anticipation was thick enough to cut with a machete. I was at total peace, but we were all aware of what the following day could hold.

Uncertainty is always the hardest part. Everyone expected great things, but we were ready for this surgery to be behind us. Of course, a six to eight hour surgery can put a damper on any evening if you think about it long and hard enough.

Dad said a prayer for my surgery, and we quickly changed the subject (Psalm 105:1–5). I enjoyed every delicious bite, taking no thought about what tomorrow would hold for me. I knew this food was better than anything I would be served on a tray during my hospital stay, so I made the most of it before my required fast. I even splurged on a decadent chocolate dessert.

My husband, Jim, is always very supportive of me and (like his father) an extremely caring man. I could see the rising concern in his bright blue eyes on the short drive back to our hotel, and I assured him that God had brought us too far to let us down now (Job 10:12). I was asleep before my head hit the pillow. I slept like a baby and awoke only to hear the sound of a rude alarm clock proclaiming the ridiculously early start of a very long day.

As a mother, I usually wake up every few hours to make sure my kids are okay. That night I didn't wake up one time, not even to roll over. I rested in a deep and uninterrupted sleep all night long, wrapping myself in a cocoon of inexplicable peace (Hebrews 13:20–21). I awoke completely refreshed, knowing that I was ready for whatever challenge my day would hold.

I had a very long list of what "not to do" before surgery.

I couldn't use any soaps or lotions, wear jewelry, apply anything scented, eat, wear makeup, or use any hair products. I must say I was not looking exceptionally attractive when I arrived with my Starbucks in hand at the surgical center bright and early with only one eye open.

I couldn't remember the last time I was up at this ungodly hour, or when the Houston traffic had ever been so light. I was anticipating a nice, long nap, knowing that my day would be over in the blink of an eye. I knew it would not flash by so quickly for family and friends gathered in the waiting room. They would be waiting the length of an entire workday for my results. I come from a long line of impatient people, so I knew this would be the ultimate test.

The hospital check-in was quick and easy. I was assigned a bed with yet another lovely blue designer hospital gown to match my monogrammed hospital bracelet. Several nurses and technicians came in with various forms of paperwork announcing that my surgery would start in a few hours, at 8:00 a.m. This was their "late" day. Lucky me.

Still, I was thrilled to be the patient and not the doctor. I was already nodding off, and they hadn't even started pumping me full of pain meds. There was no way I would be able to wake up at this insane hour on a daily basis and function with any reasonable sense, much less perform a life-saving surgery. I was not built to run at dark thirty.

I was once again reminded of the sheer dedication of this talented team of doctors and medical personnel who would be with me for the greater part of the day, as if they had nothing better to do. I prayed that God would guide their hands and honor them for saving me and prayed for blessings beyond measure for their devotion to curing a relentless disease.

The nurses came to prep me for surgery, letting me know that due to the length of my surgery, it was highly likely I would wake up in Intensive Care. Nothing need go wrong for me to wake up in ICU. They did not want me to be concerned if I did not open my eyes in a regular recovery room with the other patients.

The staff was very informative and kind as they explained how my day would unfold. The only thing I did not understand was why they were so perky. It was only 6:00 a.m. for crying out loud! I began to silently pray that God would take charge of everyone who touched me that day (Psalm 109:26–27).

Nurses hooked up six slow-feeding IVs that coaxed pain killers into my system that would eventually knock me out. I was becoming goofier with every poke of the needle, hoping the words coming out of my mouth were remotely making sense and not offensive to anyone in the room. At the same time, I just didn't give a rip. Fog was coating my brain, and I knew it was only a matter of a few short moments before I would be out, sleeping like Rip Van Winkle.

As the meds slowly continued to drip, my gurney was wheeled into an enormous room the size of the bottom floor of an average home. It seemed gigantic to me on my little gurney, as huge lights flashed in my eyes, and medical personnel ran around like ants scurrying in all directions.

The anesthesiologist came over and told me they were going to use an epidural for the surgery and would leave it in for a few days until the pain subsided. I started to lean over to allow him to insert the epidural needle when he smiled at me and said, "The needle is already inserted. Just relax." I was there. He didn't have to ask me to relax because I was already headed to La-la Land.

Maybe it was the drugs, but I started to feel like a science experiment that the entire school had shown up to watch. There was a lot of commotion in the room, and my mind was the only thing moving slowly. I recognized an intern from the day before who had attended high school with my sister. I yelled out, "My sister said to tell you hello."

Of course, when you have that much valium being pumped into your system, you have no idea how loud you are. He was very kind and asked if I had talked to her the night before. I continued yelling. "Yes, she said that you were the big stud on campus in her high school." All of the doctors and nurses started snickering and making cat calls. Yes, I had unknowingly, completely humiliated this doctor in front of his peers.

I probably should have felt badly for the guy, but I didn't. The last thing I said with one final look around the room was, "This place doesn't look anything like *Grey's Anatomy*." And that was it. It was lights out for me and the end of my spectacularly educated conversation with the people who were holding my life in their hands.

It was 7:30 p.m. when I gingerly cracked my eyes open. It felt like I had just closed them only moments before. Was it really over? No one had informed me of any details yet, but my surgery had lasted over eleven and a half hours. I started scanning the room to find the sign that said ICU but found none.

Praise God! Even though my surgery was almost twice as long as anticipated, I was in a regular room!

My husband was pacing beside my bed and anxiously jiggling about a thousand dollars in change in his jeans pocket. At least it sounded like a thousand dollars in coins right next to a microphone smashing together over and over again, and he was standing right next to my ear drum.

I had no idea how long I had been there or how long the surgery had taken, but I knew that if Jim didn't stop jingling all of that change the sound would make me deaf soon. I screamed out, "Stop!" The sound coming from my mouth was a faint whisper, as the intubation tube had just been removed from my throat and I had almost no voice left.

I couldn't feel a thing. I was completely numb, and my vision was so blurred that I could not make out many of the finer details in my room. Still, when my husband looked down at me lying motionless in the bed save for my batting eyelashes, I could tell he was thrilled to see my brown eyes open. I could feel the joy and relief washing over him as the ungodly clashing sound coming from his pocket came to an abrupt halt.

It was probably the first and only time he was ever glad to hear me screaming at him. It was only then that I found out how long the surgery had taken. I had blinked away an entire day.

I could hear a man in the recovery room next to me moaning very loudly in excruciating pain. Fortunately, everything for me was still fuzzy, and soon I would lapse into another nap that would rival any hibernating bear.

At some point I was wheeled to my assigned hospital room. I had zero memory of my day. Nonetheless, an overwhelming sense of peace coated me from the inside out, telling me that during this very important day, God had completely healed me from head to toe just as he had promised the night fear tried to claim the victory in my hotel room (Matthew 15:30–31).

The next morning I woke up to visitors, my parents and aunt. At least that is what I was told. It was great to see everyone through a misty fog and know the surgery was behind me and everything had gone smoothly.

I was sitting up in my hospital bed, chatting away as if I knew how the surgery had gone or what day it was. I was blissfully floating through the clouds, trying desperately to form sentence structures that actually made sense. With six IVs and an epidural still attached to my body, it was a lot of work to talk or even blink an eye. I was still having trouble with blurry vision, so I just blinked from one person to the next, hoping that my words had some semblance of order.

Dr. Oates, my plastic surgeon, came in to talk to me about how smoothly the surgery had gone. He began to unwrap the surgical bandages covering the gigantic stump that had become the bottom half of my leg and foot. Previously Dr. Oates had warned me that it would look like they had stitched a raw steak onto my leg; and it would take several months for the new muscle to settle into its new home. So when Dr. Oates unveiled my leg, I saw that his words rang true. My lower leg was enormous. I looked at him and said, "Holy God! Please tell me that bad boy is going to shrink in time."

My leg had morphed into yet another irregular and hideous shape. My ankle was larger than my kneecap, and stitches poked up from every possible angle—from the inside, from the outside, from layers in between. I felt like Raggedy Ann. If one of the stitches gave way, would my entire foot fall off? In between stitches was every possible color of the rainbow, a culmination of bruising versus the discoloration caused by weeks of radiation. It was a sight to behold.

I immediately felt bad with the realization that the man standing before me as I perused my leg had just saved my life, and I was criticizing his handiwork. I hadn't meant to be critical, but the drugs pumping through my body were like truth serum. I didn't think about much before it flew out of my mouth. I was so grateful for Dr. Oates's help, but I was hoping that my right leg was not going to weigh twice as much as it had before and remain a giant discolored mass.

Dr. Oates quickly assured me that the re-located muscle and tissue would settle down into my leg, and over the next year it would shift back to a normal size. If after this time I was not satisfied with the shape of my leg, Dr. Oates said he would go back in and pare down the muscle to fit my shin perfectly. I smiled at him and thanked him for spending the day with me and my fat leg.

The first two days after surgery were a complete blank. And when I say complete blank, I mean if my life depended on it, I could not tell you what I said or did. I had been told before the surgery that the nurses were going to keep two to three IVs in my arm for antibiotics, pain killers, and any type of emergency that arose until my discharge.

By the end of the second day, the epidural inserted before surgery was still in my back. These extra-strength pain meds were being pumped into my lower body at a numbing rate, and my legs felt like they weighed a ton. The epidural was supposed to be in my back for about five days, but I was doing so well that I requested it be removed the day after surgery, which was a welcome relief. My brain could form a complete thought now in under half an hour. I almost sounded intelligent.

Next came the allergic reactions to the medications. This was always exciting. Some of the antibiotics and pain meds were too strong for me, so my body reacted shortly after they dripped down from my IV. Once again I felt like my lungs were collapsing and I couldn't breathe. I was having bad flashbacks of my emergency room episode, so I asked my mom to open the Bible and read from Psalms 61.

After the first severe reaction I requested oral medications on demand only. No more massive drips.

When the nurse came in with pills, I would take one, not two. That was enough to make the pain tolerable. Since I wasn't putting any pressure on my ankle and the bandages were too big to change the position of my leg in the bed, I was fine. I wanted to have semi-coherent conversations with my surgeons when they came to my room bright and early each morning to check on my progress. Even though my mom was somewhere in my hospital room taking mental notes, I wanted to remember what the doctors were telling me and be able to ask questions that were beyond a second grade level.

When the meds weren't making me crazy, the constant attention from the nurses was about to push me over the edge. For the first five days after the surgery, the plastic surgeon ordered the nurses to come in every hour on the hour to check my leg and make sure the skin and muscle grafts were adhering and healing correctly. If either of the grafts started to show a lack of blood flowing underneath the skin flap, the surgery would have to be re-done immediately, regardless of the hour.

If there was no blood flow at 2:00 a.m., the nurses were

ordered to call the surgeon to come back in and completely re-do the entire eleven and a half-hour surgery with new body parts. I was hoping a third surgery was not in my immediate future.

So all day, and all night, the nurses would throw on the lights, invariably drop my cell phone off the side table, smashing it on the floor, take my vitals, and check my skin flap to make sure there was a heartbeat underneath. I was amazed at how quickly the doctors could find the heartbeat in the light of day and how long it took the nurses in the middle of the night.

I was not allowed to get out of bed for seven days for any reason. If I moved my foot the wrong way and the skin flap ripped or moved in the wrong direction, the surgery would have to be re-done. I just wanted to go to the potty by myself or take a shower and wash my hair. I wanted to shave my legs (or actually my one good leg) and wash my own face. These were not options. You don't realize how much the little things in life mean until you cannot get out of bed for five seconds.

By the fifth day I was totally exhausted, and my "nice" was wearing thin. I wanted to sleep for more than fifty minutes before someone came in to my room, turned on every possible light, and asked me questions I was no longer interested in answering. I wanted to sleep, uninterrupted, for about two weeks.

When the doctor came in for my daily checkup, I let him know that I would probably hurt someone very soon if I didn't get to sleep through the night. When I didn't even pretend to smile, he quickly put a keep out sign on my door. I slept like a log, and by morning I was a new person with the same bad hairdo.

At this point I was allowed to be daring and dangerous, dangling my right foot over the side of the bed to get the blood flowing in a new direction. I could not apply pressure to the leg; I could only dangle it over the side of the bed and feel the rushing blood flowing through the surgical site. The highlight of my day was doing this every few hours for fifteen minutes at a time.

I was so excited for this new exercise because I knew it would be a piece of cake. Mentally, I wanted to run the one hundred-yard dash through the hospital parking lot. Dangling my oversized leg should be a cinch.

I began this small dangling feat for fifteen minutes of sheer agony, while beads of sweat broke out on my forehead. It seemed like an eternity, and I was sure that my face was turning all shades of green while my stomach churned. Horrible nausea hit me like a tidal wave as the blood started to move through the tissue under the new skin flap for the very first time. And here I was, stuck in bed. If I had to vomit, I was going to be in big trouble.

Another day had passed, and I was ready to move on to bigger and better things like going home, cranking up my air conditioner, and sleeping in my own bed where people were smart enough not to wake me up unless the house was on fire. I didn't want anyone checking my vitals or oxygen levels or tapping on my leg. If I needed someone to break my phone in the middle of the night, I was sure my kids could do the job.

I was mentally ready to walk but had no idea how physically demanding it would be to finally pull my five-foot-two-inch self out of bed. I thought dangling my leg was hard work, but actually hoisting it out of bed and putting it to good use gave whole new meaning to excruciating pain. My leg weighed four thousand pounds when I was finally allowed to roll over and slide off my hospital bed.

I felt as if the fattest man in the world were sitting on my lap. My leg was nothing more than dead weight, like a slab of meat that just would not move no matter what signals my brain sent out. Unfortunately, the signals I was receiving loud and clear said that the process was going to take much longer than I had originally anticipated.

Finally, my big day came. The technician arrived with my very own shiny new walker. I felt like a senior citizen on my way to the early bird lunch special. I started laughing when he came in because the walker was enormous and came up to my armpits. I asked if he had any walkers for pygmies, or if he could possibly steal one from the pediatric ward. He smiled and left the oversized walker in my room. Eventually the physical therapist came in and was able to find a smaller one in the children's wing.

I was finally off to the races, so excited to be out of bed that I was sure they would have to order another EKG at any moment! This was my big chance to show the doctors that I was ready to shower and hit the road. They could start filling out the paperwork to spring me from this joint.

As these lofty aspirations flooded my mind, I began to inch toward the door with all the gusto I could muster. Every cell was straining from the energy exertion. I was probably burning three thousand calories a minute. It took me what seemed like a day and a half to reach the doorway of my room, but I made it. Perhaps I had overestimated my physical abilities just a tad in my zeal to head home.

The physical therapist guided me toward a small circular pathway leading around the nurses' station and back to my room. I made it about one third of the way around the nurses' station before exhaustion claimed me, and I began to break out in a sweat in the middle of an air-conditioned room. I felt like I had run the Boston Marathon, and severe pain was racking my leg from top to bottom. My right leg was like exceptionally heavy jello that I had absolutely no control over.

I wanted to get back in bed again and find my remote. I couldn't believe it. Here was my big chance to walk, and I was blowing it. I was out of bed for less than ten minutes, and I was begging to get back in between my soft cotton sheets and rest my leg. What a wimp!

Just about this time, my doctors came in, and I was sure that they were going to extend my stay, as I obviously couldn't get myself out of a burning building. While my mind was clouded with the hard work that lay ahead, my doctors had come to give me the good news from the surgery I had just put behind me. The pathology reports were complete. There were no remaining cancer cells in my body. I was officially cancer free!

I wanted to scream and thank God for this amazing act of love (Joel 2:25–27). I wanted to let everyone around me know that God had done it again (Isaiah 61:1–3). I was healed!

To hear my doctors come into my hospital room and medically confirm the cancer was gone was an overwhelming and inexplicable sensation as gratitude consumed the very core of my being. It was the sweetest and most enormous victory of my life, as God's promise to me became reality. It was a feeling of total triumph of good over evil. I was speechless as the tears began to pour down my face once again (Psalm 108: 1–6, 12–13).

If I could have gotten out of bed on my own without falling flat on my face, I would have danced on my one good leg. I would have run up to the doctors and wrapped my arms around them in gratitude. They had given me their all for that one day, October 18, 2006. They had not given up due to the late hour or the complexity of the surgery. And now I would live for many, many days to come.

I was grateful, blessed, and highly favored. It just doesn't get any better than that (Psalm 33:18–22).

All IVs and drainage tubes were removed, and I was released after what seemed like an emotional and physical eternity on October 25, 2006. In reality, it took only one week of my life to confirm the surgery results. The nurses wheeled me out to my mom's car, and I breathed in the most refreshingly clean air of my life. Today was the first day of my newly-constructed life.

My doctors ordered me to spend the night in Houston to ensure that I had no trouble functioning on my own in the real world. I was psyched to spend a night without the constant attention of the nursing staff and looking forward to eating a dinner that wasn't served on a tray and did not include Ensure.

I now had the luxury of wearing real clothes that covered both my front and back, and enjoying a wonderfully hot, steaming shower all by myself. As long as my showers were quick and my leg was somewhat elevated and covered with a plastic sleeve, there was no pain involved, only glorious relief at washing away days worth of grime.

After a delicious plate of Mexican food, I slept for eight full hours on a comfy couch with no lights flashing in my eyes, no blood pressure machines, no oxygen check, no thermometers, no "how are you feeling today?" I was in heaven.

When I awoke the next morning, I felt like a champ.

I was ready for the short drive home to see my girls. I was ready to be a wife and mom again. I was ready to tell everyone who would listen about God's amazing mercy that had saved my life in just one day (Isaiah 12:2–6).

Promises Fulfilled

The miles passed quickly from Houston to San Antonio. I was home, I was whole, and I was cancer free. It was really, really good to be me!

I have been blessed to visit many beautiful places and meet wonderful people from all walks of life, but there was no exotic sandy beach on earth that could rival the beauty of my home in that moment. There was nowhere I would rather have been. If the president had invited me to the White House for dinner, I would have gladly turned him down just to watch my barefooted girls running full speed ahead toward the car. The breath I didn't even know I was holding was released as joy flooded my soul at the sweetest sight on earth.

I gingerly lifted my enormous, ceramic-encased leg out of the car and onto my driveway. Grabbing the walker from the seat behind me, I slowly and painfully inched my way to the house with my kids tagging along, trying to hurry me along the sidewalk (Deuteronomy 6:5–9). They wanted to show me all of the great artwork they had made just for my homecoming.

It was all I could do to not break down in the middle of

my yard and sob with the realization that my nightmare was fading, and my sadness was turning to sheer joy.

> I will extol you, O Lord, for you have lifted me up, and have not let my foes rejoice over me. O Lord my God, I cried out to you, and you healed me. O Lord, you brought my soul up from the grave; you have kept me alive, that I should not go down to the pit. Sing praise to the Lord, you saints of his, and give thanks at the remembrance of his holy name. For his anger is but for a moment, his favor is for life; weeping may endure for the night, but joy comes in the morning. You have turned for me my mourning into dancing; you have put off my sackcloth and clothed me with gladness, to the end that my glory may sing praise to you and not be silent. O Lord my God, I will give thanks to you forever.
>
> Psalm 30:1–5, 11–12

Here I was, just four short months after my diagnosis, and I was home. I no longer had to concern myself with how much the cancer inside me was growing before my next surgery could cut it out. It was over!

I continued making my way up the driveway to the house. Once inside, I noticed a hospital bed with brand new crisp sheets in my living room conveniently located between the TV and the bathroom. This fabulously comfortable bed made it easy to elevate my leg without twisting it and was the brainstorm of my husband and father-in-law. It was a welcome surprise.

My husband had also set up a tall table next to my bed so I could access my laptop and cell phone and get back to my life. However, I was totally exhausted on every level. My mind was going a million miles an hour, and my body was telling me it was naptime. I was allowed to get out of bed for ten minutes every two hours so as not to put too much pressure on my leg or crack the delicate ceramic cast.

Not putting pressure on a leg that hurts is really not that hard. I stayed in bed and kept my leg elevated. I did not want my leg to look like an elephant forever, so I followed the doctor's orders to the letter, certain that he knew more about cosmetic surgeries than I did.

I wanted to come through with flying colors so everyone could see I was a living testimony of God's absolute mercy and grace. I expected the recovery to be extremely painful, but it wasn't anywhere close to what I had anticipated. As long as my leg was up, life was pretty good. And since I was going to be temporarily stuck in bed, I began to write in my journal. I wanted to keep track of the blessings raining down on my life so that I could share them with others who needed a small slice of hope.

People continued to ask, "Why didn't you ask why this happened to you?" My response was simple. "Why bother?" If someone who can breathe into the eye of a storm and immediately cease all churning says they are going to hold my hand and carry me through, then who am I to question them? God allowed David, a nobody shepherd boy, to pull five smooth stones from a brook and defeat a giant that an entire country was living in fear of (1 Samuel 17:40–51).

> Then David said to the Philistine, "You come to me with a sword, with a spear, and with a javelin. But I

come to you in the name of the Lord of hosts, the God
of the armies of Israel, whom you have defied. This day
the Lord will deliver you into my hand, and I will strike
you and take your head from you. And this day I will
give the carcasses of the camp of the Philistines to the
birds of the air and the wild beasts of the earth, that all
the earth may know that there is a God in Israel. Then
all this assembly shall know that the Lord does not save
with sword and spear; for the battle *is* the Lord's, and
he will give you into our hands."

1 Samuel 17:45–47 (emphasis added)

I was David; a complete nobody facing my own personal
giant. But I stood up to Satan and let him know I was going
to conquer this cancer. Cancer would *never* conquer me! The
God of Israel showed up just in time and restored to me the
joy of my salvation (Psalm 51:12). My life wasn't like it had
been before I was diagnosed; it was so much better in ways
that I could never have imagined.

I was smack dab in the middle of a cancer blessing. And yes,
even terminal circumstances can bless you if you allow them to.

When I first heard the words, "You have leiomyosarcoma,"
I had no idea my miracle would come in just four short months,
but I held fast to the promise God gave me in Psalm 61.

Today I have no promise that my cancer won't return at
any time with a vengeance no matter how many years go by
or how long I live. The threat of spreading and recurrence
diminishes with age but is an ever-present possibility. But I
know that my Redeemer lives. I have great faith that if God
can heal me once, he can do it again (Hebrews 11:1). What
once caused a numbing shock to chill my spine now causes

me to dance with joy at the realization that every time I share my story it gives the next person hope.

I decided that for me cancer was as simple as C.A.N.C.E.R.: Christ's Answer was Nailed to the Cross and Earned my Redemption.

From the very beginning, I thanked God for his provision. I thanked him for loving me just like I am. I thanked him for sending his son to die for me. I thanked him all day, every day. When my eyes opened in the morning, I thanked him (Colossians 3:15–17). When my eyes closed at night, I thanked him.

On one hand, I had great faith that with God on my team, I could weather any storm. On the other hand, I knew that whatever measure of grace or mercy was awarded me, it was completely without merit. I was unworthy of even asking for a pardon from this cancer death sentence, yet my Creator had granted me a full pardon from an incurable and ruthless disease.

Not-so-Random
Acts of Kindness

Having my leg re-constructed was an enormous undertaking, so I braced myself for a tedious and painful recovery. I wasn't worried. I just knew it would take awhile. As is true much of the time, the anticipation was worse than the reality. The worst part of my recovery was not being allowed to do many things for myself and only walking a few brief minutes each day. I was turning into a couch potato, as every time I tried to move it took an enormous amount of time and energy.

Each evening as I encased myself in the comfort of over-stuffed pillows and fresh sheets in the hospital bed located in my living room, the blessings would begin to flow over me all over again. In the morning I would wake up and have to re-bandage and treat my leg. My three-year-old daughter thought it was a great game to play doctor and help me put my "wrapper" on my leg each day. She thought she was Dr. House from TV.

My right leg was not ready for any real pressure or exercise, so this meant that cooking and housework were not in the cards for me. My kids were not looking forward to skipping any meals, so I knew we would have to put together an alternate plan. Once again God met my need and shocked me with his goodness. Having already received so many enormous blessings, I didn't expect any more to come my way, but the blessing parade continued.

My friend Syndie orchestrated a plan for meals to be delivered to my house (Matthew 6:1–4). I was completely overwhelmed by the sheer number of people who turned up to help by bringing us lunch, dinner, dessert, volunteer to watch our kids, mow the lawn, do the dishes, bathe our dogs, help with the laundry, you name it. There was a volunteer for every possible household chore (Romans 13:8–10).

From the day I returned from Houston after my marathon surgery, friends and church members alike began bringing enormous quantities of delicious food for my family. For six weeks this non-stop parade of multi-course meals and desserts continued to fill our home. In my life I had seen many acts of kindness but had never witnessed a more genuine and touching outpouring of love (Luke 6:38).

These men and women weren't bringing hamburgers from the local drive-thru; they were bringing homemade meals, desserts, toys for my kids, books and magazines for me, and delicious apple pie for my husband. They would stay long enough to let me know they were praying for me and then head out the door (Matthew 25:35–40). It seemed there were just a few minutes between the time one guest would leave and the doorbell would ring. It was as if I could hear God whispering, "I love you, Tish," with each ringing of the bell. Each person who walked through my door ministered to me in a way I didn't even know was possible.

Syndie stayed one afternoon to help color my hair. Dr. Pauli, my pediatrician, came to give me a flu shot so I wouldn't get sick during the winter with my radiated immune system. He also brought a pizza. My dentist sent teeth whitener along with the food. Another friend, Maureen, sent candles and joke books with a colorful belt. Dr. Colbert sent vitamins and health magazines. Many people sent healthy snacks and homemade goodies.

People I didn't even know sent bags of incredibly thoughtful items like DVDs, chapstick, puzzles, books, and things to help occupy my time while I couldn't get out of bed. There were flowers, fruit, cookies and an assortment of just about everything that can be delivered to your front door. Every evening I expected the circus to come to a grinding halt, understanding that all of these people surely had better things to do. Every morning I would receive another call asking how I was doing and when was a good time to come by with something new.

After a few weeks, I graduated from a walker for ten minutes every two hours to a full-time wheelchair with an extension to elevate my leg. I was getting pretty good at wheeling myself around when my plastic surgeon, Dr. Oates, broke the news that it was time to get up and start walking.

Dr. Oates began encouraging me to start walking around the block. I really love Dr. Oates. He is an exceptionally brilliant and kind man, but I was very clear with him when it came to my new exercise regimen. I was neither an outdoor person nor an athlete before my surgery and wasn't planning on becoming one now. I had no intention of walking around my block. There was no air condition outside, and we were in the middle of a Texas summer. He said, "Go walk at the mall." Like I said, I love Dr. Oates.

I didn't actually go to the mall, knowing this might just be the straw that broke my husband's back. So, I started walking around my own living room, just a little more each day. Dr. Oates and I struck a mutual compromise. If I would start exercising on my own, I would not have to return to Houston for physical therapy. I would have stood on my head eight hours a day to not have to leave my kids for another six weeks, so I was off to the races right in my very own living room.

It was exhausting walking again. What an enormous chore! I didn't recall being short of breath from walking before. I felt like I had a yacht tied to my waist that I had to physically drag off the dock just to get out of bed. I decided to stay inside my house where it was safe in case I fell, since my leg was nothing more than dead weight at this point.

I remember vividly trying to help my kids learn how to walk, and I was pretty sure they were better at it as babies than I was after my surgery. I was wobbly. I was in pain, and I just wanted to press a button to make my muscle shrink into place and start working. I looked like a baby grabbing every guardrail or piece of furniture in my path to keep from falling on my rear.

By November 13, 2006, I headed back to work to find some new home loans and immerse myself in my normal, hectic work week. I wanted to keep working for hours on end, talking to customers and acting like I didn't just have an eleven-and-a-half-hour surgery. I soon found out that it's not really a good idea to quote loan rates when your brain is concentrating on the pain in your body.

Regaining my strength was going to be a battle all its own, as my body was just plain worn out. My mind was racing in every possible direction, telling me that I had a million things on my "to do" list, and my body was at a standstill. My leg was throbbing.

I had to stop. I was simply out of gas. I could no longer keep going on just a few hours of sleep a night like I did in the weeks prior to my surgery when I was cramming a month's worth of errands into one week. My body needed lots of rest to function. My bionic leg was healing from the inside out, with enough stitches to make a formal gown. I was faced with the realization that being cancer free didn't mean that my body was going to suddenly snap back to my pre-diagnosis, pre-surgery state.

As much as I wanted to run my life at full speed, it just wasn't going to happen. It would take several months to get back to any sense of normalcy and for the swelling to decrease. After a year, if my leg still looked grotesquely huge, like the pillar of an antebellum mansion, then the plastic surgeon could cut it down and make sure that it fit more snugly in my bone structure.

It was slow going for a while, but I was in this for the long haul, so I started pacing myself. I knew that there would never come a day in my life where I decided I just didn't want to walk. It wasn't like I was going to wake up one day and not need my legs. It was time to face reality and get off my butt and exercise—a word I have despised since birth. I wanted to get my leg in good enough shape to last me for the next sixty-five years.

I walked as long as I could, which initially was just a few labored steps that got me around the living room and over to the coffee table to grab the TV remote. On a really ambitious day I could make it to the fridge and get a drink. The first few weeks it didn't take long for my leg to give out, and then it was time to stop and return to the safety of the couch cushions.

I wasn't going to push myself to extreme limits, but I wanted to make enough progress on my own to avoid physical therapy at the hospital.

So, even though I enjoy exercising second only to walking over hot coals, I was doing it. My children were a constant, living reminder of what I had to lose. I had been given a second lease on life, and I was exceptionally grateful for that, even if it meant I had to get up and walk on my giant, excessively heavy leg that made me walk like Pirate Pete. All I needed to complete my look was a parrot on my shoulder, as I certainly looked like someone who had recently walked the plank in shark-infested waters.

A Time for Thanksgiving

The girls were out of school and the office was closed. It was the time of year where everyone sits around the table with family and friends to eat at one sitting more than Jenny Craig would allow in a month. It was time to don the stretchy pants and sit around the table and enjoy the laughter of small cousins playing together once again. Most importantly, it was the annual day to give thanks. What could be better than that? It was time to give thanks for the whirlwind ride that was my life in 2006.

Every year my family gathers at the ranch to spend time together eating and thanking God for all that he has done in our lives, for we are truly blessed (Psalm 34:1). If he never does another thing for us, we have already been blessed beyond measure (Psalm 115:1). This year I couldn't make the trip because I was physically exhausted and didn't think my leg would last that many hours in a car with small children.

I hated to miss the ranch but knew that if my recovery didn't go well, the repercussions would last a lifetime. I could miss one Thanksgiving gathering, but I didn't want to miss celebrating the greatest Thanksgiving of my life (Psalm 100). God had blessed me beyond my ability to comprehend and certainly beyond my deserving. Giving thanks to him for saving my life was a must. First Chronicles 16:34 says, "Oh, give thanks to the Lord, for he is good! For his mercy endures forever."

Normally, after a delicious, home-cooked Thanksgiving lunch with all the traditional trimmings, we gather as a family in the lodge at the ranch to thank God for his blessings in our lives (Psalm 96:1–4).

I did not want to miss out on verbally proclaiming the unparalleled blessings that God had bestowed upon me that year, so I sent an email to be read aloud. The email succinctly stated a very simple message. I was alive only because of the unmerited grace of God, and every fiber of my being was grateful. I thanked each family member for the role they played in supporting me through my illness, treatment, and recovery.

Each of my relatives had carved out a piece of every day since my diagnosis to lift my case before the throne of God, and I wanted them to know on this very special day, in this very special year of healing, that their love and support had not gone unnoticed.

I absolutely without a doubt could not have done it without the constant love and relentless support of my friends and family (Psalm 34:4–10). They never asked me how horrible it was; they just prayed for me and smiled. Each friend or family member had taken a piece of my burden, a piece of my sorrow, a piece of my fear, a piece of my sickness, and carried it for me. I had very little to carry on my own, for a burden shared is certainly much lighter.

One family holiday blended into the next. I blinked and it was Christmas. This time of year for most Americans is typically chaotic and busy with frantic shopping, party planning, church cantatas, and numerous tedious end-of-the-year activities that can be maddening. This year I made a pact with myself to take Christmas slower and enjoy. I was going to breathe in every bit of goodness that the holiday offered.

I was up and around more and able to stay awake past lunch. I no longer needed pain killers and was able to walk very well on my leg without assistance and without breaking into a sweat every time I even thought about walking.

I returned to M.D. Anderson for a post-surgery checkup, and the swelling was down considerably. My doctors were elated at what they were calling a quick recovery. Were they kidding? Quick for whom? Quick as opposed to the time it took to build the Eiffel Tower? I had been on the other end of this phenomenally large leg for weeks now and didn't feel like time was just flying by as I was dragging this bad boy around my house.

One sweet nurse couldn't believe that I had not attended one physical therapy session at the hospital. I told her that God had been very good to me, and when she asked me what type of cancer I had, she said, "Yes ma'am, he sure has been good to you. I see a lot of sarcomas in this building, but almost all of them come to physical therapy. I cannot believe how well your leg is healing." I smiled and said, "It's just a God thing because I'm allergic to exercise."

I didn't have an elephant leg anymore. My leg had both skin and muscle grafts on it, but all was functioning very well and seemingly ahead of schedule. I wasn't doing the one hundred-yard dash, but I was able to do the things I needed to do in the normal course of a day. My surgical scars that extended from the top of my thigh to the bottom of my right leg were healing well, the massive amount of stitches had been removed, and the days of being bed ridden were becoming a distant memory.

The kindness and dedication of the doctors who continue to treat me never leave my thoughts. They are my heroes. They helped to give two precious girls their mother back. Actually, they gave them back a new and improved mother. I pray God rains tremendous blessings on their lives for all they did for me and my family (Romans 13:7).

Much to Celebrate!

2007 started off with a bang. I was beginning a brand new year with a clean slate and an insatiable joy that radiated from every part of my new life. On New Year's Eve it is our family tradition to gather at church around midnight and pray in the New Year. This year it was especially important for me to attend, even if my children slept through the entire service on our church pew.

When it was my turn to pray in the family circle, tears of sheer gratitude and joy flooded my cheeks. My body shook as I stammered out words that did not come close to conveying how I felt. But God looks on the heart, so I knew that he understood (1 Samuel 16:7). How do you thank God for sparing your life, for healing you from a rare and incurable disease?

Everyone in our family thanked God for my healing, for his mercy on us, and for his continued outpouring of blessings. In 2007 God had shown up and showed off in an enormous way! I had won the greatest lotto ever, and I didn't even have to buy a ticket. I felt like the richest person alive. I had been given a priceless gift that could not have been purchased with any amount of money (Matthew 13:45–46).

If Bill Gates had filled the back of my Suburban with cash, he could not have blessed me with a fraction of the intensity that God had indulged me with over my four-month cancer journey. My healing could not have been earned. It was a gift. I not only learned but lived to find out that the ultimate luxury is a great life. I will never again take that for granted.

I asked God to send those people to me who were sailing in their own personal Titanic adventure and needed encouragement (Psalm 66:8–12, 16).

I knew that if I didn't share my story with those facing a similar battle, my healing was in vain. God healed me to help others, to demonstrate to others that he is the great physician, and to offer them hope. He healed me so I could be a better wife and mother, so I could do my small part to make my community a better place (Psalm 103:1–4). And I didn't have to look very far to find that there were many more people than I wanted to know about battling cancer and other terminal diseases, dealing with other life-altering circumstances. It seemed like everywhere I turned someone else was telling me their own heart-wrenching story.

These people were sick with every serious ailment known to man. They had suddenly lost a loved one. They were missing an arm or leg due to disease or illness. They were young. They were old. They were still in the trenches looking like deer in the headlights, wondering what to do. Some were weary from the fight and ready to wave a white flag. Some were leading victorious lives and relishing each day. Many were consumed by fear.

Those fighting cancer started coming out of the woodwork, asking about my own personal struggles and looking for a granule of hope. I couldn't open my email without finding another prayer request or plea for help. Had I been living in a cave, or was there a sudden surge of people battling cancer? I was laminated with bad news on every side. When I asked God to send me those in need, he certainly honored my request.

I was grateful for the opportunity to reach out to them. I was grateful that we could speak the same language, the language of hope and healing, the language of deep angst and absolute heart break. Had I not walked through that cancer valley, I could not have begun to understand their very unique and all-consuming circumstances.

I would not have understood that when you hear the word cancer attached to your name, everything else immediately hits the back burner of life. If you are having financial troubles, does it matter if you can't pay your bills when you're dead? If you don't like your job, you can't work if you don't wake up because your treatment wasn't effective.

I had been given this extraordinary opportunity to reach out to a diverse community that was comprised of members from every possible demographic. No one was exempt from the Cancer Club. I was not going to be the exception to the rule. I was unexpectedly and irrevocably a card-carrying member for life, and I could not have felt more blessed.

Cancer had only been a speed bump in my life. It was a bump that temporarily slowed down my ride but did not even put a dent in my fender. Wax on. Wax off. I was ready to look around and smell the roses. I was ready to reach out more than ever but knew I had to clean up everything in my own life before I could truly help others (Luke 10:29–37).

I mean, how can one get the log out of their own eye when they are busy checking out someone else's splinters? It was time for me to shed not only the shoes I didn't need but to take my journey one step further.

I began cleaning out my relationship closet to rid my life of those precious souls who constantly played the role of the victim or constantly needed negative attention and continually drained everyone in their path—those who thrived on self-imposed drama. These are the people who don't want to truly overcome anything, because if they did, they would need a personality transplant. Generally these people deceive themselves into thinking they are just so fantastic to be around, and just about the last breath of perfection left on earth.

I was done with perfection. I wanted people who weren't afraid to admit their faults and lay them at the cross. I wanted crooked pots and crooked lids. I rid myself of these perfect Christians in a very succinct manner, letting them know that since our values were obviously very different, I wished them the very best, but it was time for us to part ways.

It was unbelievably liberating. I couldn't believe how much time and energy I had left over to spend on the people I actually liked. My life was becoming more enjoyable by the second.

I began to pray even harder for God to expose those things I needed to change within myself. Prayers are like million dollar checks. A check has no value until you cash it. A prayer has no value until you pray it (Philippians 4:6–7). There is so much power in prayer it is scary (Matthew 9:6–8).

I would pray about something, and it would happen

almost immediately, or the thing I didn't want to give up didn't matter to me anymore. There were greater things at stake in my new universe, which was now suffering from a total realignment of priorities. I wanted to make sure that my life was completely in tune with the Word of God so that no weapon formed against me would prosper (Isaiah 54:17).

My dad always says, "Don't tell me you love me; show me." I wanted to show God how much I loved him. I wanted my life to honor him in every possible way. I wanted people to see him through me and to experience random acts of kindness by what God was doing through me (Matthew 5:16).

The more I prayed, the more my world evolved into a supernaturally perfect place for me. Not that I am a perfect person by any stretch of the imagination (just ask my siblings or husband), but I was right where God wanted me to be. When you are spiritually exactly where God wants you, there is no greater or more satisfying place on earth. God turns on his fountain of blessings, and you feel like you are drowning in goodness and mercy.

Once you know this feeling, you never want to do anything to offend God because you don't want the outpouring of goodness to stop. Favor is addictive in all the right ways.

On February 3, 2007, I turned thirty-eight. It was another red letter day. It was a day that Satan told me many times I would never see. When I awoke that morning, the house was silent, but in my mind there was a huge parade going on in my honor. Jesus was right there, leading my parade and winking at me as if I never had a thing to fear because I was in the palm of his hand the entire time. I was shouting praises for his unmerited mercy and grace.

It was a true victory for my whole family and for many others who had prayed and fasted for me for months during my treatment, surgery, and recovery (Matthew 17:20–21).

Of course, Satan never likes us to celebrate God's goodness in our lives.

My next check-up at M.D. Anderson showed a "shadow" on my MRI. Was it some type of infection in my leg again? It looked like it was in the bone. Was it just a shadow from where my foot had moved during the test? It didn't look like a cancer recurrence, but the cells gave the doctors cause for concern. That did not excite me one bit. The oncologist asked me to come back in six to eight weeks for further examination and to inspect how the infection or "shadow" was manifesting itself. They would compare those tests with what they were looking at today to see if there was cause for alarm.

Are you kidding me? Come back in six to eight weeks to find out what we need to do? Can't we just do something now? I'm already here. How about giving me a shot just in case it is some type of infection? How about scheduling another surgery to scrape it out so we can test it and find out right away what this "shadow" really is?

Am I really waiting again to find out if my leg is infected one more time? Could it be another staph infection? That was just a real thrill a minute. How much infection can one leg take? Will this affect the outcome of my surgery? Will I have to re-live another eleven-and-a-half-hour surgery? Can I find out something today before I leave instead of waiting another two months for an update?

God has such a great sense of humor, and I usually do too, but when we're talking about another infection in my leg or a possible recurrence of cancer, I wasn't really ready to chill out and sit idly by, hoping that another tumor wasn't manifesting itself. I knew that Satan would try to use this time to plant seeds of fear in my mind, and I could not allow that to happen.

I didn't want to take the wait and see approach (Psalm 102:1–2). I wanted the microwave approach. Press a button, and thirty seconds later my problem was solved. I don't like waiting for the water in my shower to get hot, and I certainly didn't want to wait eight weeks to find out what the "shadow" in my MRI really was and if there was cause for concern. I wanted to know right then and there. Of course, that wasn't going to happen. I would wait ten weeks before finding out that it was indeed scar tissue and no cancer was anywhere in my body; no bone was infected. The surgery had been a total success.

The Hits Just Keep Coming

During the week of July 4, 2007, I was back at the hospital emergency room in San Antonio. It seemed I could not get enough of the hospital scene, the fabulous cafeteria food, and the uber comfy and very fashionable blue scrubs.

This time I was admitted with my four-year-old daughter, Kassidee, just days before her fifth birthday. She had inexplicable swelling, was covered with a rash, and her test results baffled the doctors. They thought she might have been bitten by a brown recluse spider, might have cat scratch fever, might have some strep with scarlet fever and some staph infection. This is a lot for a body that weighs less than fifty pounds.

The first day we were in the hospital was non-stop testing with x-rays, blood tests, and an MRI. The MRI results were sent to the surgeon around midnight, and he immediately drove to the hospital to examine our precious baby girl. He arrived with a nurse in tow to take Kassidee directly to the operating room.

The MRI showed that Kassidee had been diagnosed with necrotizing fasceitis, a bacterial flesh-eating virus. The surgeon had come into her room to rush her to surgery and cut off the majority of her arm and chest, then graft it back together using her other body parts. Again, I couldn't believe my ears. But I could not allow the numbness to consume me, because my daughter's life was on the line.

Now I knew what the mothers at M.D. Anderson felt like when their small child was being rolled on a gurney down the hospital corridor. The realization made my heart ache to the point of bursting.

I started praying immediately. The surgeon asked about Kassidee's symptoms and said that what he saw on her body was pink living flesh with no signs of decay or abscess, which was in direct contradiction to the MRI report.

Kassi was sent to ICU for antibiotics and was to report to surgery first thing in the morning to remove the affected tissue; it was only a matter of time before a major reconstructive surgery was performed on my tiny toddler.

We began calling family and friends to get every prayer warrior on their knees (1 Thessalonians 5:17–18). My dad had just been admitted to the hospital while we were in the emergency room. Was there no end to this health crisis? I was warmin' up my boots to kick Satan one more time. It is one thing to attack me, and it is something entirely different to attack my child. I was incensed! Satan was going down. I turned on the tape player in Kassidee's ICU room and played healing scriptures all night long. If Satan wanted to get my attention, he had it. Now I was ready to turn a little unwanted attention back his way.

I began calling my individual family members with this latest report of cutting my child's arm and chest tissue off and grafting muscles from her leg, only to find that every one of my sibling's children were sick with some sort of fever, virus, or sudden illness. We were all sick at the same time, so none of us could do very much to help the other except pray.

So we prayed for ourselves and for one another. Never in the history of our family had everyone been sick at once. It was the Lalapalooza of sickness. Everyone was on their own stage with a different set of symptoms, and the hits just kept coming. But God showed up in spades.

The following morning when the pediatric surgeon showed up to determine the extent of the surgery Kassidee would need and the amount of tissue he would be cutting off, he was amazed at how her skin was still pink and not decaying or "crunchy." There was no medical explanation as to why she would be able to keep her chubby little arm. But God.

The doctors and nurses were still going to keep her under close observation and isolation as she had an infectious disease. This meant that she was allowed no visitors, and the staff members coming in to see her often wore lovely plastic Hazmat suits which were very comforting for a small child. Not.

But Kassidee is a fighter, and she did not shed one tear during the many, many hours of constant testing, needle poking, or just plain feeling bad. The blood tests were relentless and given night and day, but she did not complain once.

The tests continued, and so did the swelling. The swelling was increasing across her chest and down her arm, but her pink skin was not dying. The test results showed nothing out of the ordinary, but the naked eye could tell that there was something terribly wrong.

Again, there were so many reasons for us to be thankful. There was never a time when Kassidee was afraid or nervous. She was insanely sick but continued to play with small toys and draw pictures in her hospital bed while she was hooked up to various machines monitoring her every move, inside and out.

> The Lord is my light and my salvation; whom shall I fear? The Lord is the strength of my life; of whom shall I be afraid? When the wicked come against me to eat up my flesh, my enemies and foes, they stumbled and fell... For in the time of trouble He shall hide me in his pavilion; in the secret place of His tabernacle He shall hide me; He shall set me high upon a rock... Hear, O Lord, when I cry with my voice! Have mercy also upon me, and answer me... I would have lost heart, unless I had believed that I would see the goodness of the Lord in the land of the living.
>
> Psalm 27:1, 2, 5, 7, 13

I began to read Psalm 27 to Kassidee. Even though she was too small to understand what was happening to her, I wanted to invite the Holy Spirit into her room (Psalm 51:10–12). We were once again in need of a visit from the Great Physician. And I needed to set a tone of complete calm in her room so that she did not pick up on the severity of her illness. Again, I was grateful that she was much too young to understand the gravity of the situation.

An infectious disease doctor was called in. Even though it was a holiday, she immediately came in on the 4th of July after reading Kassidee's MRI report. Like the surgeon before her, the infectious disease doctor examined Kassidee and was happy to see her tiny arm looked much better than the report stated. She told us, "To be honest with you, my last patient with symptoms lesser than these expired."

The words registered in my brain quickly, but we had been through so many life-altering illnesses lately and sailed through with flying colors on the wings of grace that I knew this would be no exception. Without wasting a second, I looked up and smiled, telling the doctor in no uncertain terms, "God healed me from cancer this year, and we are expecting great things for Kassidee as well (1 Peter 3:15)." When she asked the type of cancer I had, I told her. She frowned and said, "Wow, that's a bad one." My response was simple. "We serve a big God."

As I watched the doctor leave Kassidee's hospital room, I felt a sweet weight crushing me. At that exact moment I began to fully absorb how deeply God's love and mercy had entrenched my entire family, even down to the smallest member (Mark 10:14–15). I knew we had far surpassed our allotted mercy limit, but he just kept pouring it on (Psalm 34:19–20).

Our pediatrician, Dr. Pauli, was working some major overtime with every one of our kids down at the same time. He was up at the hospital early with me, at the office with my siblings, and back at night to see how our day had progressed. The man needed some roller skates to keep up with the insanity in my family, and a whole lot of caffeine.

We are all immensely grateful for the constant blessing Dr. Pauli is in our lives and love the fact that he prays over our kids when they are sick. I am amazed that he has not put our phone numbers on call blocker yet. He continues to help us day and night as our kids arrive at his home on his days off for a quick exam or to call in a prescription. He truly is one of the greatest blessings my children have ever known on earth.

That week of sheer craziness, Kassidee was diagnosed with several different things beyond the necrotizing fasceitis, such as staph, an internal strep, and a high likelihood of a brown recluse spider bite. The tests continued night and day for the better part of a week, as Kassi's outward healthy appearance didn't match the lab results. Her blood work remained perfect, though there was not a square inch of porcelain skin on her body that was left unbruised.

Much to the doctor's surprise, there was no infection in her bone. Even after these numerous tests were conducted over and over again to confirm the diagnoses, Kassidee never had one surgery. Not one cut or one stitch (Psalm 120:1).

Initially the emergency room doctor said it was likely Kassidee would be in the hospital for four to six weeks with an extensive recovery upon release. She stayed in the hospital for five days. That was a long and miraculous road for her tiny body to travel in such a short period of time, but we knew once again that only God's mercy had granted this miraculous and speedy recovery.

My four-year-old was going home with some serious medications, but she still had her arm. There was no permanent damage or decaying skin. She would be home in time for her fifth birthday, and it was time to pull out the piñata and bask in the goodness that had surely followed Kassi throughout her hospital stay.

We were once again at home, sleeping in our own beds

and relishing the fact that no medical personnel were anywhere in site. I had not left the hospital in days, so it was a
nice change of scenery. It was also an added bonus that our
friends could now visit, and no one had to wear head-to-toe
plastic to walk in the door.

Over the course of the next two years, I would have the plea-
sure of sharing my smile with my doctors at M.D. Anderson
every three months. Every report, every test, every x-ray
continued to come back clean. With each visit to Houston, I
was becoming more and more encouraged.

Unfortunately, the little engine that could came to a slow,
grinding halt in January of 2008 when I started feeling terribly sick. I was plagued with chronic fatigue, deep depression, and insomnia. It was a lethal mix. I didn't want to go
anywhere or do anything and had to assemble a new team of
doctors in San Antonio, as Houston was too far away. I was
too tired to even think about driving there.

Once again I became a human lab rat and went through
the required battery of tests. After several months it was determined that I had severe vitamin deficiencies along with severe
auto-immune disease. My thyroid had "too many nodules to
count," and it was highly likely that they were cancerous. This
was certainly a new take on cancer for me, but somehow hearing it the second time didn't have the same sting.

I was ready for more treatment or surgery. Just point me
in the right direction and let me get rid of this all-consuming
exhaustion. Of course, the doctors wanted to make sure I was
healthy enough to go through yet another surgery. So, once

again I waited until my blood work was completed and my vitamin levels were deemed high enough to help with rapid healing. By December of 2008, I was ready for surgery.

In just over three hours, my thyroid was out, my parathyroids and lymph nodes were checked, and I was wheeled back to my hospital room for an overnight stay. I don't remember much of the first few hours after surgery, as I tried to fight through the drug-induced fog, but that evening the doctors were at my bedside giving me the great news. My thyroid was completely out, nothing left behind, and all other areas were nodule free, indicating there was no other cause for concern regarding cancer spreading. Now we just needed to wait for the pathology reports.

I was elated. This surgery was like going through the drive-through at Wendy's, short and sweet. I could get up and go to the bathroom by myself because both legs worked. I only had to spend one night in the hospital, and my vitals seemed to be holding out just fine. The night of my surgery they gave me one last pain killer, and I was ready to be released by the following morning after my delicious jell-o breakfast.

Two days after my surgery I felt more energized than I had all year long. Unfortunately, I was still holding my breath to see what the pathology report would say. I was preparing myself for the inevitable iodized radiation, as that was the recommended treatment for this type of cancer. I knew that if God had carried me through radiation once, he could take me and my fried hair through it one more time. It was like having my second baby. No big surprises.

My surgery was on Monday. By Wednesday I felt great, and on Friday afternoon my surgeon was calling with the pathology report. No malignancy. Once again my breath caught in my throat, and tears of gratitude poured down my cheeks as my very kind surgeon said, "I guess those prayers worked out for you, didn't they? But then again, they always do."

> For I know the thoughts that I think toward you, says the Lord, thoughts of peace and not of evil, to give you a future and a hope. Then you will call upon me and go and pray to me, and I will listen to you. And you will seek me and find me, when you search for me with all your heart. I will be found by you, says the Lord, and I will bring you back from your captivity; I will gather you from all the nations and from all the places where I have driven you, says the Lord, and I will bring you to the place from which I cause you to be carried away captive.
>
> Jeremiah 29:11–14

|LIVE

listen|imagine|view|experience

AUDIO BOOK DOWNLOAD INCLUDED WITH THIS BOOK!

In your hands you hold a complete digital entertainment package. Besides purchasing the paper version of this book, this book includes a free download of the audio version of this book. Simply use the code listed below when visiting our website. Once downloaded to your computer, you can listen to the book through your computer's speakers, burn it to an audio CD or save the file to your portable music device (such as Apple's popular iPod) and listen on the go!

How to get your free audio book digital download:

1. Visit www.tatepublishing.com and click on the e|LIVE logo on the home page.
2. Enter the following coupon code:
   2a0e-9c68-ca3f-a2a6-2956-41f8-9268-4568
3. Download the audio book from your e|LIVE digital locker and begin enjoying your new digital entertainment package today!